Transform Beyond the Buffet: Unraveling the Complexities of Binge Eating

Unique Kade

Table of Contents

Introduction

Unlocking the Door to Liberation

In a world often defined by excess and abundance, a silent struggle lurks behind the laughter at feasts and the clinking of glasses in celebration. This is the realm of binge eating, a complex and often misunderstood journey that countless individuals embark upon, cloaked in **shame** and **secrecy**.

Welcome to **"Transform Beyond the Buffet: Unraveling the Complexities of Binge Eating,"** a profound exploration into the depths of an enigma that touches lives across every spectrum. This is not **just** a **book**; it is an **invitation** to **break free from** the **chains** that **bind** you, an opportunity to traverse the **labyrinth** of emotions, societal pressures, and

personal battles that characterize the journey of **binge eating.**

In these pages, we delve beyond the surface, beyond the **polished** veneer of societal norms, and venture into the heart of this intricate challenge. We **confront** the stigmas, dispel the myths, and carve a **path** toward understanding and compassion. This is a **call** to **arms**, not just for those who battle binge eating but for a society that must open its eyes to the silent **struggles** endured by **many**.

Prepare to embark on a transformative odyssey where knowledge becomes a lantern, illuminating the shadows of shame. As we unravel the psychological, social, and biological threads that weave the tapestry of binge eating, we emerge with a profound understanding that paves the way for healing.

Are you ready to embark on a journey of self-discovery and liberation? The buffet of life awaits, and beyond it lies a world where you dictate the terms, not the cravings. Open the door to your liberation. Your story of triumph begins here.

Understanding the Basics

At the core of any exploration lies the necessity to comprehend the fundamentals. When it comes to binge eating, peeling back the layers to reveal its essence is crucial for you, those grappling with the disorder and the wider community seeking empathy and awareness.

The Act of Binge Eating

1. **Defining the Act:** Binge eating is not merely an indulgence; it's a rampant consumption of food within a discrete period, accompanied by a perceived loss of control. This goes beyond the usual moments of overeating during celebrations or gatherings. It is marked by a compelling urge, an almost automatic response, often in isolation, that sets it apart from everyday eating habits.

2. **Frequency and Quantity:** Understanding binge eating involves recognizing patterns. Frequency varies from person to person, some experiencing it sporadically while others struggle with more regular episodes. The quantity of food consumed during a binge can be staggering, far surpassing what one would consider a normal meal.

3. Emotional and Psychological Dimensions

4. **The Role of Emotions:** Binge eating is a dance between food and emotions, a coping mechanism for stress, anxiety, depression, or even boredom. Unraveling the emotional threads entwined with the act is crucial for understanding its roots.

5. **Loss of Control:** Central to binge eating is losing control during an episode. It's a moment where rationality surrenders to the overpowering drive to consume, creating a sense of powerlessness and guilt afterwards.

<u>Conclusion</u>

In delving into the basics of binge eating, we lay the groundwork for a more profound exploration of the disorder. By understanding the intricacies of the act, its emotional underpinnings, and its impact on mental and physical health, we pave the way for empathy, awareness, and effective avenues for support and recovery.

This is not just about recognizing the symptoms; it's about comprehending the human experience behind each bite, acknowledging the struggle, and moving towards a landscape of healing and understanding.

Differentiating Binge Eating from Other Eating Disorders

In the intricate landscape of eating disorders, each disorder is a unique expression of a complex relationship with food. Understanding binge eating requires a nuanced exploration of how it differentiates itself from other disorders, such as anorexia nervosa and bulimia nervosa.

1. Binge Eating vs. Anorexia Nervosa: The Spectrum of Control

★ **Anorexia Nervosa Overview:** Anorexia nervosa is characterized by restrictive eating, an intense fear of gaining weight, and a distorted body image. Individuals with anorexia often perceive themselves as overweight despite being underweight.

★ **Differentiation:** The fundamental contrast lies in the approach to food. While anorexia involves extreme food restriction, binge eating entails consuming large quantities of food in a short period. The motivations behind these behaviors are distinct, with anorexia rooted in fear of weight gain and a desire for control. At the same time, binge eating often stems from emotional triggers.

2. Binge Eating vs. Bulimia Nervosa: The Role of Purging

★ **Bulimia Nervosa Overview:** Bulimia nervosa involves episodes of overeating followed by compensatory behaviors such as vomiting, excessive exercise, or fasting. Like binge eating, it is characterized by a sense of loss of control during episodes.

★ **Differentiation:** The key difference lies in the post-binge behaviors. Compensatory actions do not accompany binge eating, whereas bulimia involves purging to rid the body of the consumed calories.

This crucial distinction shapes the trajectory of each disorder and influences its physical and psychological consequences.

3. Compulsive Overeating vs. Binge Eating Disorder: Clinical Definitions

★ **Compulsive Overeating Overview:** The term "compulsive overeating" is sometimes used interchangeably with binge eating. However, within clinical contexts, Binge Eating Disorder (BED) is a distinct diagnosis characterized by recurrent episodes of binge eating without regular compensatory behaviors.

★ **Differentiation:** BED is marked by a lack of control during eating episodes, a feeling of distress afterwards, and a significant impact on daily life. The clinical criteria for BED provide a framework for distinguishing between occasional overeating and a more pervasive and distressing pattern of binge eating.

4. Binge Eating's Unique Identity: The Absence of Compensatory Behaviors

★ **Defining Feature:** What sets binge eating apart is the absence of immediate compensatory actions. Unlike bulimia, there is no immediate purging, and unlike anorexia, there is no extreme caloric restriction. Binge eating stands alone, defined by the act and its emotional aftermath.

Conclusion

In unraveling the complexities of binge eating, it's paramount to appreciate the distinctions between various eating disorders. This chapter illuminates the unique features of binge eating, emphasizing its divergence from anorexia nervosa, bulimia nervosa, and even terms like compulsive overeating. Through this nuanced understanding, we not only refine our comprehension of binge eating but also lay the groundwork for targeted interventions, destigmatization, and enhanced support for those navigating the intricate web of eating disorders.

Chapter 1

The Spectrum of Binge Eating

In the vast tapestry of human experience, the journey through binge eating is neither monochromatic nor linear. Welcome to a chapter that ventures into the intricate nuances of this complex dance with consumption, emotion, and control.

As we embark on "The Spectrum of Binge Eating," envision a spectrum that refracts the light of understanding, revealing shades from the subtle to the profound and will delve deep into **Mild to Severe: Grasping the Variability.**

Mild to Severe: Grasping the Variability

Within the intricate tapestry of binge eating, a spectrum defies simplicity, weaving a narrative of diverse struggles and triumphs as we embark on the exploration of "Mild to Severe: Grasping the Variability."

Under Mild to Severe: Grasping the Variability, you will learn and dive deep into

1. Examining Different Levels of Binge Eating Severity
2. Recognizing Subtle Signs and Symptoms

Pick your pen, jot and let's dive deep into it.

Note: don't forget to practice.

Examining Different Levels of Binge Eating Severity

Binge eating, a multifaceted and often clandestine struggle, exists along a spectrum ranging from mild to severe. This section delves into the intricate nuances of this spectrum, recognizing that the experience of binge eating is not a uniform journey but a diverse landscape with varying degrees of intensity.

Understanding the Spectrum

1. *The Mild Ripples*

At the mild end of the spectrum, individuals may experience sporadic episodes of binge eating. These occurrences, while infrequent, can be significant in their impact, triggering emotions of guilt and shame. Recognizing the mild ripples involves understanding the subtle signs, such as occasional overindulgence or a pattern of emotional eating during stress.

2. *Moderate Undulations*

Moving along the spectrum, moderate levels of binge eating introduce a more regular pattern. If you are at this stage, you may find yourself grappling with a consistent struggle to control your eating habits.

The frequency of episodes increases, and emotional triggers become more pronounced. Identifying signs of moderate undulations, such as increased **preoccupation** with food and a **noticeable** loss of control during episodes, is essential.

Exploring the Depths

1. *Intensified Currents*

In the middle range of severity, binge eating intensifies, becoming a more pervasive aspect of daily life. Individuals may experience a deeper emotional connection to their episodes, with a heightened sense of distress and loss of control.

Recognizing intensified currents involves acknowledging the impact on mental well-being and understanding how binge eating may be used as a coping mechanism for underlying emotional challenges.

2. *Severe Storms*

At the severe end of the spectrum, binge eating becomes a formidable storm, dominating the landscape of an individual's existence. The frequency and intensity of episodes escalate significantly, leading to severe physical and psychological consequences.

Recognizing severe storms necessitates a keen awareness of the profound impact on mental health and overall well-being and the potential development of comorbid conditions.

Signs and Symptoms Across the Spectrum

1. Behavioral Cues

- **Mild:** Occasional overeating, especially during times of stress or emotional distress.

- **Moderate:** Regular overconsumption episodes often accompany a sense of guilt and loss of control.

- **Intensified:** More pervasive and frequent episodes with a notable impact on daily routines and activities.

- **Severe:** Compulsive and uncontrollable eating, potentially leading to isolation and withdrawal from social interactions.

2. Emotional Indicators

- **Mild:** Occasional feelings of guilt or shame following episodes.

- **Moderate:** Increasing emotional distress and preoccupation with body image and weight.

- **Intensified:** Heightened emotional turmoil, with binge eating serving as a primary coping mechanism.

- **Severe:** Overwhelming emotions of guilt, shame, and a significant negative impact on mental health.

Implications for Treatment and Support

Understanding the variability in binge eating severity is paramount for tailoring effective interventions. Treatment strategies should be nuanced, considering the unique needs of individuals at different points along the spectrum. A comprehensive approach will involve therapeutic interventions, nutritional counseling, and, in severe cases, medical support.

In conclusion, examining different levels of binge eating severity is crucial to fostering empathy, awareness, and targeted support. Recognizing the spectrum's diverse manifestations can pave the way for a more comprehensive understanding of this complex and often stigmatized struggle, ultimately fostering a more compassionate and effective approach to treatment and recovery.

Recognizing Subtle Signs and Symptoms of Binge Eating

Binge eating, with its intricate web of emotional and psychological components, often manifests through subtle signs and symptoms that can be easily overlooked. This section aims to unravel the nuanced cues, providing a comprehensive guide to recognizing the subtle indicators of binge eating allowing for early intervention and support.

1. Changes in Eating Patterns

- **Increased Secrecy:** One subtle sign of binge eating involves increased secrecy surrounding food consumption. Individuals may choose to eat in isolation, away from the eyes of others, to conceal the extent of their food intake during episodes.

- **Erratic Eating Times:** Binge eating can disrupt regular meal patterns. Recognizing subtle changes, such as frequent nighttime eating or erratic meal schedules, may indicate a struggle with binge eating.

2. Emotional and Psychological Shifts

- **Heightened Stress or Anxiety:** Binge eating often emerges as a coping mechanism for stress and anxiety. Recognizing an escalation in stress levels or the emergence of anxiety-related behaviors can be a key indicator.

- **Mood Swings:** Subtle mood swings, particularly following meals or eating episodes, may signify an emotional connection to binge eating. Individuals might experience guilt, shame, or irritability after consuming much food.

3. Changes in Social Behavior

- **Withdrawal from Social Activities:** Binge eating can lead to feelings of shame and embarrassment, prompting individuals to withdraw from social interactions that involve food. Recognizing a sudden reluctance to participate in shared meals or events may hint at underlying struggles.

- **Avoidance of Food-Related Conversations:** Individuals grappling with binge eating may subtly avoid discussing food, diets, or weight-related topics. Recognizing a shift in conversational preferences can be indicative of an ongoing struggle.

4. Physical Indicators

- **Fluctuations in Weight:** While binge eating doesn't always result in immediate weight gain, recognizing subtle fluctuations in weight can be a sign.

Individuals may engage in cycles of overeating followed by restrictive behaviors, leading to weight changes over time.

- **Evidence of Hidden Food Containers:** Subtle signs may include the discovery of hidden food wrappers or containers, indicating a desire to conceal the extent of food consumption.

5. Psychological Strain

- **Increased Self-Criticism:** Binge eating often leads to negative self-talk and heightened self-criticism. Recognizing subtle shifts in an individual's self-perception, particularly expressions of guilt or shame, can be crucial.

- **Obsessive Thoughts about Food:** An individual's preoccupation with food, recipes, or meal planning may escalate subtly. Recognizing an increase in obsessive thoughts about food may indicate an underlying struggle with binge eating.

Conclusion

Recognizing the subtle signs and symptoms of binge eating demands a keen awareness of behavioral, emotional, social, and physical indicators. By understanding these nuances, you will identify the early stages of binge eating and offer support.

Early intervention and open communication play pivotal roles in addressing binge eating, fostering a compassionate environment that encourages seeking professional help and promoting a journey towards your healing and recovery.

Chapter 2

The Psychology of Binge Eating

Welcome to a chapter that delves into the intricate realm where the mind and appetite intertwine, shaping the narrative of binge eating. In **"The Psychology of Binge Eating: Emotional Triggers,"** we unravel the threads that connect our emotions to the complex dance of consumption, exploring the profound influence of stress, anxiety, and depression on our relationship with food.

In this chapter we will dive deep into:

1. **Emotional Triggers**

    ★ Exploring Emotional Connections to Binge Eating

    ★ Stress, Anxiety, and Depression

2. **Mindfulness and Binge Eating**
> ★ Strategies for Cultivating Awareness
>
> ★ Mindful Eating Practices

In the following chapters, we embark on a voyage of self-discovery, unveiling the layers of the emotional tapestry that shroud our eating habits. "The Psychology of Binge Eating: Emotional Triggers" invites you to challenge preconceptions, explore the depths of your emotional landscape, and embrace the empowering tools of mindfulness to forge a path towards liberation from the complexities of binge eating.

Emotional Triggers

Beneath the surface of our daily lives lies an intricate dance between the heart and the plate, where emotions and eating converge in a delicate ballet.

In this section, **"Emotional Triggers,"** we embark on a journey to unmask the invisible forces that propel us towards the solace of food. This is not just an exploration of appetite; it's an odyssey through the labyrinth of our emotions, uncovering the profound influence of stress, anxiety, and depression on the tapestry of our eating habits.

In the exploration that follows, we unravel the invisible threads that tie our emotions to the act of eating. "Emotional Triggers" is an invitation to peer into the shadows, acknowledge the silent forces at play, and empower ourselves to break free from the chains of unconscious consumption.

Join me on this journey of self-discovery as we unmask the emotional triggers that shape our eating habits, paving the way for a more conscious and empowered relationship with food.

Exploring Emotional Connections to Binge Eating

Understanding binge eating extends beyond mere food consumption; it involves unraveling the intricate tapestry of emotions that intertwine with this complex behavior. In this exploration, we delve into the emotional connections to binge eating, shedding light on the psychological nuances that drive individuals towards the solace of food.

1. Emotional Triggers as Catalysts

Stress: The Weight on the Plate

Stress, an omnipresent force in modern life, often becomes a catalyst for binge eating. In times of stress, the body's response triggers a desire for comfort, and food becomes a readily available source.

Exploring the emotional connection between stress and binge eating involves recognizing stressors—be they work-related, personal, or environmental—and understanding how they become emotional triggers for impulsive consumption.

Anxiety: The Knot in the Stomach

Anxiety, with its pervasive sense of unease, intertwines with binge eating in a delicate dance. Food becomes a coping mechanism for some to soothe the relentless worry and nervous energy.

Exploring the emotional connection to anxiety involves examining the rituals and behaviors associated with eating during anxious moments and uncovering the patterns that link the emotional state to the act of bingeing.

Depression: Shadows in the Cravings

Depression casts a long shadow on the landscape of binge eating. Food may be a reprieve as you grapple with sadness, hopelessness, or emptiness. Exploring the emotional connection to depression entails understanding the role of food in alleviating emotional pain and the impact of depressive symptoms on eating behaviors.

2. The Vicious Cycle of Emotional Eating
Temporary Relief and Long-Term Consequences

Binge eating often provides a fleeting sense of relief from emotional distress, creating a cyclical pattern. Understanding this cycle involves exploring the momentary escape that food offers, juxtaposed with the long-term consequences of increased guilt, shame, and potential physical health issues.

Emotional Avoidance and Suppression

Some individuals use binge eating as a strategy to avoid or suppress overwhelming emotions. Exploring this connection requires an examination of the emotional void that food fills and avoiding facing more profound psychological challenges.

3. Mindfulness as a Compassionate Response
Cultivating Awareness of Emotional Triggers

Mindfulness emerges as a transformative tool in exploring emotional connections to binge eating. Cultivating awareness involves:

- Recognizing emotional triggers in real-time.
- Acknowledging the emotions without judgment.
- Developing a compassionate response that doesn't include impulsive consumption.

Mindful Eating Practices

In response to emotional triggers, mindful eating practices become a beacon of stability. Strategies such as savoring each bite, listening to internal hunger cues, and fostering a non-judgmental attitude towards food contribute to a more conscious and intentional approach to eating.

4. Breaking the Cycle: Strategies for Intervention

Therapeutic Approaches

Breaking the cycle of emotional eating often requires therapeutic intervention. Cognitive-behavioural therapy (CBT), Dialectical Behavior Therapy (DBT), and other therapeutic modalities offer individuals tools to explore and address the underlying emotional connections to binge eating.

Building Healthy Coping Mechanisms

Exploring alternative, healthier coping mechanisms becomes pivotal. This involves replacing impulsive eating with activities that address emotional needs, such as engaging in hobbies, exercise, or seeking support from friends and mental health professionals.

<u>Conclusion</u>

In unraveling the emotional connections to binge eating, we unveil a profound understanding of the intricate dance between emotions and eating behaviors. This exploration is not just a theoretical exercise; it's a compassionate journey towards self-awareness and healing.

By acknowledging the emotional triggers, understanding their impact, and embracing mindful approaches to eating, individuals can begin to untangle the threads that bind them to the cycle of binge eating, paving the way for a more balanced and empowered relationship with food and emotions.

Stress, Anxiety, and Depression

➢ Stress

Stress, an inevitable and pervasive facet of modern life, plays a significant role in shaping our behaviors, including our relationship with food. In this exploration, we delve into the intricate dynamics of stress and its impact on binge eating, recognizing stress as a potent emotional trigger that can lead individuals down the path of impulsive consumption.

1. Defining Stress: The Modern Dilemma

Psychological and Physiological Responses

Stress, in its essence, is the body's natural response to perceived threats or challenges. This can manifest as a psychological response, such as worry or anxiety, and a physiological response, including increased heart rate and the release of stress hormones like cortisol. Understanding stress involves recognizing its dual nature as a mental and physical phenomenon.

Types of Stress: Chronic and Acute

Stress can be classified into two main categories: chronic and acute. Acute stress is the body's immediate reaction to a perceived threat, often called the "fight or flight" response.

Chronic stress, on the other hand, is an ongoing, prolonged state of stress that can result from persistent life challenges, such as work pressures or relationship issues.

2. Stress and Binge Eating: Unraveling the Connection

Coping Mechanisms and Comfort Eating

One of the most prevalent responses to stress is adopting coping mechanisms; for many, this involves turning to food for comfort.

Stress-induced binge eating becomes a way to self-soothe, providing a temporary escape from the pressures of daily life. Understanding the connection between stress and binge eating requires a nuanced examination of how food becomes a coping mechanism during challenging times.

The Role of Cortisol: A Biological Link

Cortisol, the primary stress hormone, is pivotal in the stress-eating connection. Elevated cortisol levels can stimulate appetite and cravings, particularly for foods high in sugar and fat. Exploring the impact of cortisol on eating behaviors unveils the intricate biological mechanisms at play during stressful situations.

3. Recognizing Stressors: Identifying Emotional Triggers

<u>Work-Related Stress</u>

Work-related stress is a common trigger for binge eating. The pressures of deadlines, performance expectations, and workplace dynamics can contribute to heightened stress levels, prompting individuals to seek solace in food.

<u>Relationship Stress</u>

Challenges in personal relationships can be potent stressors. Conflicts, breakups, or interpersonal tensions can lead individuals to turn to binge eating as a means of emotional coping.

Financial Stress

Economic uncertainties and financial pressures can induce chronic stress, impacting both mental well-being and eating behaviors. Understanding the connection between financial stress and binge eating involves exploring how monetary concerns contribute to emotional distress.

4. Breaking the Cycle: Strategies for Coping with Stress

Mindfulness and Stress Reduction Techniques

Mindfulness practices, including meditation and deep breathing exercises, offer effective tools for stress reduction. Cultivating mindfulness can interrupt the automatic response of turning to food during stressful moments.

Healthy Coping Mechanisms

Encouraging the adoption of healthy coping mechanisms is crucial in breaking the cycle of stress-induced binge eating. Engaging in regular exercise, seeking social support, and practicing self-care are essential strategies for building resilience in the face of stress.

5.   Professional   Support: Therapeutic Approaches

<u>Cognitive-Behavioral Therapy (CBT)</u>

CBT is a therapeutic approach that helps individuals identify and modify dysfunctional thought patterns and behaviors. In the context of stress and binge eating, CBT can be a valuable tool for developing healthier coping mechanisms.

<u>Mindfulness-Based Stress Reduction (MBSR)</u>

MBSR programs focus on incorporating mindfulness techniques to manage stress. These programs can equip individuals with the skills to respond to stressors without resorting to impulsive eating.

Conclusion

Understanding stress and its impact on binge eating involves a comprehensive exploration of the intricate interplay between emotional triggers, physiological responses, and coping mechanisms.

By recognizing stress as a potent influencer of eating behaviors, individuals can take proactive steps to cultivate healthier coping strategies, breaking the cycle of stress-induced binge eating.

Whether through mindfulness practices, adopting healthy coping mechanisms, or seeking professional support, the journey towards a balanced relationship with stress and food is a transformative endeavor, paving the way for improved well-being and emotional resilience.

Anxiety

Anxiety, a pervasive emotional state characterized by apprehension and fear, has profound implications for our behaviors, particularly in the realm of eating habits. This exploration delves into the intricate dynamics of anxiety and its impact on binge eating, unraveling the connections between heightened stress levels, emotional triggers, and impulsive consumption.

1. Defining Anxiety: The Complex Emotional Landscape

Generalized Anxiety Disorder (GAD)

Anxiety is a natural stress response, but when it becomes chronic and disproportionate to the perceived threat, it may manifest as Generalized Anxiety Disorder (GAD). Understanding anxiety involves recognizing its diverse manifestations, from general worries to specific phobias and its potential to shape daily behaviors.

Physiological Responses to Anxiety

Physiologically, anxiety activates the body's "fight or flight" response, releasing stress hormones like cortisol and adrenaline. These physiological changes can influence appetite, cravings, and eating patterns. Exploring anxiety entails acknowledging its dual nature as both a psychological and physiological phenomenon.

2. Anxiety and Binge Eating: Unraveling the Intricacies

<u>The Role of Emotional Eating</u>

Anxiety often triggers emotional eating, a phenomenon where individuals turn to food as a coping mechanism for emotional distress. Understanding the connection between anxiety and binge eating requires exploring how food becomes a source of comfort and distraction during anxious moments.

<u>Perfectionism and Control</u>

Individuals with anxiety may exhibit perfectionistic tendencies, seeking a sense of control in their lives. Binge eating can emerge as a way to regain control temporarily, creating a cycle where anxiety triggers the behavior, and binge eating provide a momentary escape.

3. Recognizing Anxiety Triggers: Identifying Emotional Catalysts

Social Anxiety

Social situations can act as potent triggers for anxiety. The fear of judgment or scrutiny may lead individuals to cope with social anxiety through binge eating as a way to manage uncomfortable emotions.

Performance Anxiety

In academic or professional settings, anxiety about performance and meeting expectations can contribute to emotional distress. Binge eating may serve as a coping mechanism to alleviate the pressure associated with performance anxiety.

Existential Anxiety

Existential concerns about the meaning and purpose of life can generate anxiety. Binge eating may temporarily distract from existential questions, providing a sense of immediate pleasure and comfort.

4. Breaking the Cycle: Coping Strategies for Anxiety-Induced Binge Eating

Mindfulness and Anxiety Reduction Techniques

Mindfulness practices, including meditation and mindful breathing, offer effective tools for managing anxiety. By cultivating awareness of the present moment, individuals can interrupt the automatic response of turning to food during anxious episodes.

Cognitive-Behavioral Therapy (CBT)

CBT, a widely utilized therapeutic approach, addresses maladaptive thought patterns and behaviors associated with anxiety. In the context of anxiety-induced binge eating, CBT can empower individuals to reframe negative thought patterns and develop healthier coping strategies.

5. Building Emotional Resilience: Healthy Coping Mechanisms

Regular Exercise

Physical activity is a powerful tool for managing anxiety. Exercise releases endorphins, the body's natural stress relievers, and provides a constructive outlet for anxiety-associated pent-up energy.

Social Support Networks

Building and maintaining supportive social connections can be instrumental in managing anxiety. Friends and family can provide understanding, encouragement, and companionship during challenging times.

Conclusion

Understanding anxiety and its influence on binge eating requires a holistic exploration of the emotional, psychological, and physiological dimensions of this complex relationship. By recognizing anxiety as a potential catalyst for impulsive eating, individuals can embark on a journey of self-discovery, adopting mindfulness practices, seeking therapeutic support, and cultivating healthier coping mechanisms.

The path to breaking the cycle of anxiety-induced binge eating is transformative, fostering emotional resilience and paving the way for a more balanced and empowered relationship with food and anxiety.

Depression

Depression, a pervasive mental health condition characterized by persistent feelings of sadness and loss of interest, can profoundly influence various aspects of an individual's life, including eating behaviors. This exploration delves into the intricate dynamics of depression and its impact on binge eating, unraveling the connections between emotional distress, coping mechanisms, and impulsive consumption.

1. Defining Depression: Navigating the Emotional Abyss

Major Depressive Disorder (MDD)

Depression is often diagnosed as Major Depressive Disorder (MDD) when symptoms persist for an extended period, significantly impacting daily functioning. Understanding depression involves recognizing its multifaceted nature, encompassing emotional, cognitive, and physical dimensions.

The Neurochemical Basis of Depression

Depression is associated with alterations in neurotransmitter levels, particularly serotonin, dopamine, and norepinephrine. These imbalances can impact mood, appetite, and sleep patterns, contributing to changes in eating behaviors. Exploring depression necessitates an awareness of both its emotional toll and its physiological underpinnings.

2. Depression and Binge Eating: Unraveling the Intricacies

Emotional Numbing and Comfort Eating

Individuals experiencing depression may engage in binge eating as a form of emotional numbing or seeking comfort. Food becomes a temporary escape from the persistent feelings of emptiness and despair. Understanding the connection between depression and binge eating involves exploring how food provides solace in times of emotional distress.

Lack of Motivation and Energy

Depression often manifests as profound fatigue and a lack of motivation. Binge eating may respond to these feelings, temporarily providing energy and pleasure. The exploration of depression's impact on binge eating includes understanding the role of fatigue and lethargy in shaping eating behaviors.

3. Recognizing Depression Triggers: Identifying Emotional Catalysts

Social Isolation and Loneliness

Depression can lead to social withdrawal and isolation. Feelings of loneliness may trigger binge eating as individuals attempt to cope with the void created by a lack of social connections.

Hopelessness and Helplessness

Feelings of hopelessness and helplessness, common in depression, can contribute to emotional distress. Binge eating may serve as a way to regain a sense of control and momentarily alleviate these overwhelming emotions.

Body Image Concerns

Depression can distort perceptions of self-worth and body image. Binge eating may be linked to a desire for temporary relief from negative self-perceptions or a means of self-soothing.

4. Breaking the Cycle: Coping Strategies for Depression-Induced Binge Eating

Therapeutic Approaches:
Cognitive-Behavioral Therapy (CBT) and Interpersonal Therapy (IPT)

CBT addresses negative thought patterns and behaviors associated with depression. IPT focuses on improving interpersonal relationships and communication. Both therapies can help individuals develop healthier coping mechanisms and break the cycle of depression-induced binge eating.

Medication Management

In cases of severe depression, medications such as selective serotonin reuptake inhibitors

(SSRIs) or tricyclic antidepressants may be prescribed. Medication, when combined with therapy, can help alleviate depressive symptoms and mitigate their impact on eating behaviors.

5. Building Emotional Resilience: Holistic Approaches

Regular Exercise

Exercise has been shown to positively affect mood by releasing endorphins, the body's natural mood enhancers. Engaging in regular physical activity can be an effective strategy for managing depressive symptoms and reducing the likelihood of binge eating.

Mindfulness and Meditation

Mindfulness practices, including meditation and mindful eating, offer tools for managing depressive symptoms. Cultivating present-moment awareness can interrupt automatic responses, such as turning to food in emotional distress.

Conclusion

Understanding depression and its influence on binge eating is an intricate journey that involves acknowledging the profound emotional and physiological impact of this mental health condition.

By recognizing depression as a potential catalyst for impulsive eating, individuals can embark on a path toward healing, adopting therapeutic interventions, medication management, and holistic approaches to build emotional resilience.

Breaking the cycle of depression-induced binge eating is transformative, fostering emotional well-being and opening avenues for a more balanced and empowered relationship with food and mental health.

Mindfulness and Binge Eating

In the hustle and bustle of modern life, where every demand demands our attention, mindfulness emerges as a sanctuary. This tranquil pause invites us to be fully present. In the realm of binge eating, where emotions often drive behaviors, this chapter embarks on a journey into the profound connection between mindfulness and breaking free from the cycle of impulsive consumption.

"Mindfulness and Binge Eating" is not just a guide but a journey into the essence of self-awareness, a pilgrimage toward breaking free from the chains of unconscious consumption. As we navigate the landscapes of the mindful mind, let us uncover the serenity within, forging a path toward a more balanced and empowered relationship with both food and the present moment.

Strategies for Cultivating Awareness in Binge Eating Recovery

Cultivating awareness is a cornerstone of breaking free from the cycle of binge eating. In this exploration, we delve into strategies that empower individuals to be present, to tune into their thoughts and emotions without judgment, and to forge a path towards a more mindful relationship with food.

1. Mindful Eating Practices: Nourishing the Body and Soul

Savoring Each Bite

Mindful eating involves savoring each bite with intention and attention. Encouraging individuals to engage their senses—tasting, smelling, feeling the textures—creates a heightened awareness of the eating experience. This practice shifts the focus from mere consumption to a conscious appreciation of the nourishment provided by each morsel.

Eating Without Distractions

Modern life often encourages multitasking, even during meals. However, cultivating awareness requires a departure from distractions. Encouraging individuals to eat without the interference of electronic devices or external stimuli promotes a deeper connection with eating and its associated sensations.

2. Journaling: Unveiling Patterns and Emotions

Food Diary Exploration

Keeping a food diary serves as a powerful tool for self-reflection. Recording what is eaten and the emotions, circumstances, and thoughts surrounding each meal unveils patterns and triggers. Journaling becomes a mirror, reflecting the complex interplay between emotions and eating habits.

Emotional Logging

In tandem with food diaries, emotional logging encourages individuals to delve into the emotional landscape of eating. Identifying and naming emotions associated with specific eating episodes fosters a deeper understanding of the emotional triggers that may lead to binge eating.

3. Mindfulness Meditation: Grounding in the Present Moment

Breath Awareness Meditation

Breath awareness meditation is a foundational practice in mindfulness. Focusing on the breath grounds individuals in the present moment. In the context of binge eating recovery, this practice becomes a lifeline—an anchor that individuals can return to when faced with the turbulence of emotional triggers.

Body Scan Meditation

Body scan meditation involves a systematic, mindful exploration of each part of the body. This practice heightens body awareness and helps individuals connect with physical sensations, fostering a deeper understanding of how emotions manifest physically and how they may influence eating behaviors.

4. Cognitive-Behavioural Techniques: Restructuring Thought Patterns

Thought Records

Cognitive-Behavioral Therapy (CBT) techniques, such as thought records, encourage individuals to identify and challenge negative thought patterns associated with binge eating. This strategy involves examining the accuracy and validity of thoughts, fostering a more balanced perspective.

Behavioral Chain Analysis

Behavioral chain analysis in CBT helps individuals trace the events leading to binge eating episodes. Individuals can identify specific points where mindfulness interventions can disrupt the cycle by dissecting the chain of thoughts, emotions, and behaviours.

5. Mindful Movement: Integrating Body and Mind

Yoga and Tai Chi

Mindful movement practices like yoga and Tai Chi integrate physical activity with mindfulness. These practices emphasize awareness of body sensations, breath, and movement. Incorporating mindful movement into a routine promotes a holistic approach to well-being, addressing both physical and emotional aspects.

Walking Meditation

Walking meditation shifts mindfulness from a stationary practice to one in motion. Encouraging individuals to walk with deliberate awareness fosters a connection with the body and the environment. This practice particularly benefits those who find solace in movement and struggle with sedentary mindfulness practices.

6. Professional Support: Therapeutic Guidance

Mindfulness-Based Therapies

Mindfulness-based therapies, such as Mindfulness-Based Stress Reduction (MBSR) or Mindfulness-Based Cognitive Therapy (MBCT), provide structured guidance. These therapeutic modalities offer a curriculum of mindfulness practices and strategies tailored to individuals recovering from binge eating.

Individual or Group Therapy

Professional support through individual or group therapy allows individuals to explore mindfulness in a therapeutic setting. Therapists can guide the integration of mindfulness into daily life, addressing specific challenges and tailoring strategies to individual needs.

Conclusion

Strategies for cultivating awareness in binge eating recovery are diverse, offering individuals a toolkit to navigate the complex terrain of emotions, thoughts, and behaviors. Whether through mindful eating practices, journaling, meditation, cognitive-behavioral techniques, mindful movement, or professional support, these strategies empower individuals to break free from the automaticity of binge eating and foster a conscious, mindful approach to their relationship with food and emotions. In embracing these strategies, individuals embark on a transformative journey toward self-awareness, resilience, and a balanced connection with their bodies and minds.

Mindful Eating Practices: Nourishing the Body and Soul

Mindful eating is more than a dietary approach; it's a way of engaging with food that transforms the act of nourishment into a profound and intentional experience. In this exploration, we delve into mindful eating practices that invite individuals to savor each bite, cultivate awareness, and break free from the cycle of impulsive consumption.

1. Savoring Each Bite with Intention

<u>Engaging the Senses</u>

Mindful eating begins with engaging the senses. Encouraging individuals to truly see, smell, touch, and appreciate food's visual and sensory aspects fosters a deeper connection with the eating experience. Individuals shift from mechanical eating to a more intentional and pleasurable encounter by involving the senses.

<u>Appreciating Textures and Flavors</u>

Mindful eaters focus on the textures and flavors of each bite. This practice involves paying attention to the crunch, the smoothness, the temperature, and the subtle nuances of taste. By appreciating the sensory aspects of food, individuals derive more satisfaction from each mouthful, reducing the urge to consume impulsively.

2. Eating Without Distractions

<u>Turning Off Electronics</u>

Modern life often encourages multitasking, even during meals—mindful eating advocates for turning off electronic devices and eliminating distractions. By sitting down without the interference of screens or external stimuli, individuals can fully concentrate on eating, promoting a deeper connection with their food and internal cues.

<u>Creating a Dedicated Eating Environment</u>

Establishing a dedicated eating environment fosters mindfulness. Encouraging individuals to eat at a set table, with minimal distractions, transforms meals into a ritual. This separation from chaotic surroundings allows for a focused, intentional eating experience.

3. Mindful Chewing and Swallowing

<u>Chewing Mindfully</u>

Mindful eating involves chewing each bite deliberately and thoroughly. This practice not only aids digestion but also extends the duration of the meal, allowing individuals to recognize feelings of fullness more accurately. Mindful chewing promotes a mindful pace, preventing hurried consumption.

Conscious Swallowing

Conscious swallowing is an often overlooked aspect of mindful eating. Encouraging individuals to be aware of the entire process, from chewing to swallowing, brings attention to the journey of each bite. This heightened awareness helps distinguish between physical hunger and the impulse to eat for emotional reasons.

4. Eating with Gratitude and Awareness

Expressing Gratitude

Mindful eating involves expressing gratitude for the food on the plate. Reflecting on the effort that went into producing the meal, from farming to preparation, fosters a sense of appreciation. Gratitude enhances the eating experience and encourages a mindful acknowledgment of the nourishment provided.

Listening to Internal Hunger and Fullness Cues

Practicing mindfulness includes listening to internal cues of hunger and fullness. Tuning into the body's signals helps individuals recognize when they are genuinely hungry and when they've satisfied their appetite. This awareness prevents overeating and supports a more balanced approach to nourishment.

5. Developing a Mindful Eating Ritual

Mindful Meal Beginnings

Creating a ritual around the beginning of a meal establishes a transition from daily activities to a mindful eating state. This could involve a moment of silence, a brief expression of gratitude, or taking a few deep breaths before starting the meal.

Pausing Between Bites

Encouraging individuals to pause briefly between bites introduces rhythm to the eating process. This pause provides time to assess satiety levels and appreciate the act of nourishment, preventing automatic, rapid eating.

6. Mindful Reflection After Eating

Reflection on Satisfaction

Mindful eating extends beyond the last bite. It includes reflection on satisfaction and contentment after finishing a meal. This practice involves acknowledging the nourishment received and recognizing when the body is comfortably satiated.

Awareness of Emotional Responses

Mindful reflection encompasses an awareness of emotional responses to the meal. Identifying any emotional triggers or lingering stressors helps individuals understand the connection between emotions and eating, promoting a mindful approach to emotional well-being.

Conclusion

Mindful eating practices offer a holistic approach to breaking free from impulsive consumption, providing individuals with a toolkit to foster awareness and appreciation for nourishing the body. Individuals embark on a transformative journey towards a more conscious and balanced relationship with food by savouring each bite, eliminating distractions, and developing mindful eating rituals. These practices enhance the eating experience and contribute to overall well-being, promoting a mindful approach to nourishment that extends far beyond the dining table.

Chapter 3

Social and Cultural Influences

Step into the complex weave of societal threads that shape our relationship with food. In this chapter, **"Social and Cultural Influences,"** we navigate the intricate dance between individual choices and the external forces that mold them. From the media's powerful impact on body image to the diverse perspectives on food ingrained in cultural tapestries, we unravel society's profound role in the intricate narrative of binge eating. Join us as we dissect the influence of societal pressures, media messages, and cultural norms, revealing the nuanced interplay between external environments and personal eating behaviors.

In this chapter we are going to dive into,

1. **The Role of Society in Binge Eating**

   ★ Media, Body Image, and Societal Pressures

   ★ Cultural Perspectives on Food and Eating

The Role of Society in Binge Eating

Navigating External Influences

Beyond the individual, society weaves a silent narrative that shapes our perceptions, choices, and relationships with food. In this exploration, we delve into the profound influence of societal structures on binge eating behaviors. Join us as we unravel the threads connecting societal norms, expectations, and pressures to the intricate tapestry of binge eating, shedding light on the external forces that sculpt our most intimate act—nourishing ourselves.

Media, Body Image, and Societal Pressures

→ <u>Media</u>

With its pervasive reach, media holds power to shape perceptions, influence behaviors, and define societal norms. In the context of binge eating, the impact of media on body image, self-esteem, and eating habits is profound and complex. This exploration delves into the multifaceted ways in which media contributes to the landscape of binge eating behaviors.

1. **Body Image Portrayals: The Photoshop Effect**

   <u>**Idealized Standards**</u>

Media often perpetuates idealized standards of beauty, featuring images of thinness and perfection that are often unattainable. This portrayal sets unrealistic expectations, fostering body dissatisfaction and, in some cases, triggering binge eating as individuals attempt to cope with the gap between reality and societal ideals.

The Photoshop Phenomenon

The prevalence of photo editing tools in media creates a distorted perception of beauty. Images that undergo extensive retouching contribute to a culture of comparison, where individuals may feel inadequate or dissatisfied with their bodies, potentially leading to emotional distress and maladaptive eating behaviors.

2. Diet Culture and Weight Stigma

Promotion of Dieting Trends

Media frequently promotes dieting trends, emphasizing rapid weight loss and transformation narratives. The constant influx of these messages can contribute to a diet culture that may foster an unhealthy relationship with food, encouraging extreme behaviors that can lead to binge eating episodes.

Weight Stigma and Shame

The media's portrayal of certain body types as ideal can result in weight stigma, creating a culture where individuals feel shame or judgment based on their appearance. This weight-based discrimination can be a significant emotional trigger, prompting binge eating as a way to cope with societal scrutiny.

3. Advertising and Food Marketing

Hyperpalatable Food Promotion

Food advertising often features hyper-palatable, highly processed foods rich in sugars and fats.

The constant exposure to these tempting images can stimulate cravings and impulsive eating behaviors, contributing to the development or exacerbation of binge eating habits.

Portrayal of Emotional Eating

Media representations may normalize emotional eating as a response to stress, sadness, or celebration. This normalization can influence individuals to turn to food as a coping mechanism for emotional distress, potentially contributing to the development of binge eating patterns.

4. Social Media and Peer Comparisons

The Impact of Social Media Influencers

Social media platforms, dominated by influencers, can perpetuate unrealistic body standards. Comparisons to these digitally curated images may lead to feelings of inadequacy and, in turn, contribute to emotional eating or binge episodes as individuals seek solace or distraction.

Community Narratives and Support

Conversely, social media can also be a source of support and community. Shared experiences and narratives of recovery from binge eating can foster understanding and reduce isolation, offering a counterbalance to the negative influences prevalent in traditional media.

5. Media Literacy and Empowerment

Promoting Critical Media Consumption

Empowering individuals with media literacy skills is crucial. Encouraging critical evaluation of media messages, questioning unrealistic portrayals, and fostering awareness of the persuasive techniques used in advertising can help individuals navigate media influence more effectively.

Building Resilience and Self-Esteem

Developing resilience against media pressures involves cultivating a positive self-image and self-esteem. Emphasizing diverse representations of beauty, promoting body positivity, and highlighting personal strengths can buffer individuals against the negative impact of media on their body image and eating behaviors.

Conclusion

Media plays a pivotal role in shaping societal attitudes, norms, and individual behaviors, including those related to binge eating. Recognizing the influence of media on body image, diet culture, and emotional triggers is essential for individuals seeking to navigate a healthier relationship with food. By fostering media literacy, promoting positive representations, and building resilience, individuals can reclaim agency over their narratives, mitigating the potential negative impact of media on their journey toward balanced and mindful eating.

→ __Body Image__

Body image, the subjective picture individuals hold of their bodies, is a profound and intricate aspect of human identity. In the context of binge eating, body image can play a pivotal role in shaping emotions, behaviors, and overall well-being. This exploration delves into the multifaceted nature of body image, examining its origins, societal influences, and the intricate relationship between body perception and binge eating.

1. **Origins of Body Image: Shaping Self-Perception**

   __Developmental Influences__

Body image takes shape early in life through genetic, environmental, and social factors. Childhood experiences, family dynamics, and societal influences contribute to forming body image, laying the groundwork for attitudes and perceptions that can persist into adulthood.

Cultural and Societal Standards

Cultural ideals of beauty, often perpetuated by media and societal norms, significantly influence body image. The pursuit of an "ideal" body shape or size, as dictated by prevailing cultural standards, can lead to body dissatisfaction and emotional distress, potentially triggering or exacerbating binge eating behaviors.

2. Impact of Media on Body Image

Idealized Standards and Photoshop Realities

By portraying idealized beauty standards, the media contributes to developing unrealistic body ideals. The prevalence of digitally altered images further distorts perceptions, fostering a culture of comparison and dissatisfaction that may contribute to emotional triggers for binge eating.

Diet Culture and Weight Stigma

Media's promotion of diet culture and the stigmatization of certain body sizes can significantly impact body image. Individuals may internalize societal judgments, leading to feelings of shame or inadequacy based on their appearance, potentially influencing their relationship with food and contributing to binge eating patterns.

3. Psychological Dimensions of Body Image

Body Dysmorphic Concerns

Body dysmorphic concerns involve a distorted perception of one's appearance, often accompanied by obsessive thoughts about perceived flaws. Individuals experiencing body dysmorphic tendencies may be particularly vulnerable to developing unhealthy eating behaviors, including binge eating, as they seek to cope with their distorted body image.

Self-Esteem and Self-Worth

Body image is intricately linked to self-esteem and self-worth. Negative perceptions of one's body can contribute to diminished self-esteem, fostering a cycle where individuals may turn to food as a coping mechanism to manage feelings of inadequacy or low self-worth.

4. Intersectionality and Diverse Body Experiences

Cultural Perspectives on Beauty

Diverse cultural perspectives on beauty influence individual body image experiences. Cultural norms and expectations regarding body size and shape can impact how individuals perceive themselves, shaping their attitudes toward their bodies and influencing their relationship with food.

Gender and Body Image

Gender norms and societal expectations regarding body ideals differ across genders. Understanding the unique pressures and expectations placed on individuals based on their gender is crucial in unraveling the complex dynamics of body image and its potential links to binge eating.

5. Building a Positive Body Image: Strategies and Interventions

Promoting Self-Compassion

Encouraging self-compassion involves fostering a kind and understanding relationship with one's body. Embracing imperfections and appreciating the body's body and resilience can contribute to a more positive body image, reducing the likelihood of using food as a coping mechanism.

Media Literacy and Critical Evaluation

Equipping individuals with media literacy skills enables them to evaluate and challenge unrealistic portrayals of beauty critically. By recognizing the persuasive techniques used in advertising and media, individuals can develop a more discerning approach, reducing the impact of external influences on their body image.

Counseling and Therapeutic Support

Professional counseling and therapeutic support can be invaluable in addressing negative body image and its potential links to binge eating. Therapeutic approaches, such as cognitive-behavioral therapy (CBT) and body-positive counseling, provide individuals with tools to challenge distorted perceptions and cultivate a healthier relationship with their bodies.

Conclusion

Body image, a multifaceted aspect of individual identity, holds significant implications for emotional well-being and eating behaviors, including binge eating. Recognizing the intricate interplay between societal influences, psychological dimensions, and diverse body experiences is crucial for individuals seeking to cultivate a positive body image. By promoting self-compassion, fostering media literacy, and seeking therapeutic support, individuals can embark on a transformative journey toward a more balanced, empowered, and positive relationship with their bodies and food.

→ <u>Societal Pressures</u>

Societal pressures, encompassing a myriad of expectations, norms, and cultural standards, profoundly influence individual behaviors, particularly in eating habits. This exploration delves into the intricate tapestry of societal pressures, unraveling how external expectations and cultural ideals contribute to the complex landscape of binge eating behaviors.

1. Cultural Ideals and Body Image Expectations

The Pursuit of "Ideal" Body Standards

Societal pressures often dictate an "ideal" body size and shape, perpetuated through cultural norms and media representations. The relentless pursuit of these ideals creates an environment where individuals feel compelled to conform, potentially leading to body dissatisfaction, low self-esteem, and emotional triggers that contribute to binge eating.

Body Shaming and Weight Stigma

Weight-based discrimination and body shaming are pervasive societal issues. Individuals who do not conform to societal body ideals may experience stigma and judgment, leading to feelings of shame and inadequacy. Coping with such negative societal perceptions can be challenging and may contribute to maladaptive eating behaviors, including binge eating.

2. Diet Culture and Food Morality

The Pervasiveness of Diet Culture

Diet culture, reinforced by societal pressures, promotes the idea that certain foods are "good" or "bad" and that one's worth is tied to dietary choices. This binary approach to food morality can create a fraught relationship with eating, potentially triggering binge episodes as individuals grapple with feelings of guilt or shame associated with their food choices.

The Moralization of Eating Behaviors

Societal pressures extend to moral judgments about eating behaviors. Labels such as "overeating" or "lack of willpower" may be applied to individuals, fostering a sense of moral failure. The internalization of these judgments can contribute to emotional distress, potentially leading to binge eating as a way to cope with negative emotions.

3. Social Comparison and Influences

The Impact of Social Comparison

Social comparison, exacerbated by social media, can intensify societal pressures. Constant exposure to curated images and lifestyles may make individuals compare themselves unfavorably, fostering feelings of inadequacy or needing to conform to perceived societal norms. This pressure to measure up can contribute to emotional distress and binge eating as a coping mechanism.

Peer and Family Expectations

Expectations from peers and family members play a significant role in shaping behavior.

Societal pressures to conform to familial or peer-driven expectations regarding appearance, lifestyle, or eating habits can create internal conflicts, potentially contributing to binge eating as individuals navigate the tension between societal expectations and personal autonomy.

4. Gendered Expectations and Roles

Societal Ideals and Gender Norms

Societal pressures often prescribe specific ideals and norms based on gender. The expectations of individuals to conform to these gendered standards may influence body image and eating behaviors. Gender-specific pressures can contribute to emotional distress, body dissatisfaction, and the development or exacerbation of binge eating patterns.

The Intersection of Identity and Societal Pressures

For individuals at the intersection of various identities, such as race, ethnicity, gender, and sexuality, societal pressures may be compounded. The intersectionality of identity introduces additional layers of expectations and norms that can impact body image and eating behaviors, potentially influencing the manifestation of binge eating.

5. Resilience and Coping Strategies

<u>**Building Resilience Against Societal Pressures**</u>

Building resilience involves developing strategies to withstand societal pressures and fostering a sense of self-worth independent of external expectations. Emphasizing individual strengths, cultivating a positive self-image, and surrounding oneself with supportive communities can contribute to resilience against societal influences that may contribute to binge eating.

Coping Mechanisms Beyond Food

Encouraging the development of healthy coping mechanisms beyond food is essential. Individuals can explore alternative outlets for managing stress, anxiety, or emotional distress, reducing reliance on binge eating as a primary coping strategy. This may involve engaging in creative pursuits, physical activities, or seeking professional support.

Conclusion

Societal pressures, manifested through cultural ideals, body expectations, and gender norms, intricately shape the landscape of individual behaviors, including binge eating. Recognizing the impact of these external influences is a crucial step in navigating a healthier relationship with food. By fostering resilience, challenging societal expectations, and seeking supportive communities, individuals can reclaim agency over their narratives, fostering a balanced and empowered approach to their bodies and eating behaviors.

Cultural Perspectives on Food and Eating

→ Cultural Perspectives on Food

Food is more than sustenance; it is a cultural artifact, a symbol of heritage, and a conduit for shared traditions. Exploring cultural perspectives on food, we uncover how societies conceptualize, prepare, and consume meals. This exploration delves into the profound influence of cultural norms, traditions, and values on individuals' relationships with food, shedding light on how cultural perspectives contribute to the complex landscape of eating behaviors, including binge eating.

1. **The Symbolism of Food in Culture**

Cultural Significance of Meals

In various cultures, meals are not just a means of satisfying hunger; they carry symbolic weight, often serving as expressions of identity, hospitality, and celebration. Understanding the cultural significance of different foods and eating rituals is essential in grasping the intricate relationship individuals have with the act of nourishment.

Rituals and Festivities

Cultural perspectives on food are often intertwined with rituals and festivities. Traditional meals prepared during specific ceremonies or celebrations are laden with cultural meaning, reinforcing a sense of community and shared identity. However, these cultural practices may also contribute to complex relationships with food, potentially influencing binge eating behaviors.

2. Cultural Norms and Dietary Patterns

Diversity in Dietary Habits

Cultural norms play a pivotal role in shaping dietary habits. The types of foods consumed, meal structures, and dietary restrictions are often deeply rooted in cultural traditions. While these norms contribute to culinary diversity, they can also influence individuals' perceptions of what is considered "normal" or acceptable in terms of eating behaviors.

Impact of Migration and Acculturation

For individuals navigating multiple cultural identities, the clash between traditional dietary norms and those of a new environment can create unique challenges. The process of acculturation, where individuals adopt elements of a new culture, may impact eating behaviors, potentially contributing to stress and emotional triggers for binge eating.

3. Cultural Influences on Body Image

Idealized Beauty Standards Across Cultures

Cultural perspectives on beauty ideals vary globally. In some cultures, specific body sizes or shapes may be idealized, influencing individuals' perceptions of their bodies. The internalization of these cultural ideals can contribute to body dissatisfaction, potentially triggering emotional distress and maladaptive eating behaviors, including binge eating.

Cultural Narratives and Gender Roles

Cultural expectations regarding gender roles can influence body image. Some cultures may prescribe specific ideals for men and women, impacting how individuals perceive and relate to their bodies. The intersection of cultural expectations and body image can contribute to the development of disordered eating patterns.

4. The Role of Food in Socialization

Communal Dining Traditions

In many cultures, meals are communal, fostering social bonds and a sense of belonging. Shared meals provide opportunities for connection, communication, and the reinforcement of cultural values. However, the communal nature of dining may also contribute to normalising certain eating behaviors, potentially influencing binge eating within social contexts.

Cultural Influence on Social Pressure

Cultural perspectives can shape social expectations related to food. Individuals may experience pressure to conform to cultural norms during communal meals, potentially leading to emotional distress and maladaptive eating behaviors as they navigate societal food consumption expectations.

5. Cultural Narratives and Mental Health

Stigma and Mental Health in Cultural Context

Cultural perspectives can influence the stigma associated with mental health, including disordered eating. In some cultures, mental health issues may carry a higher degree of stigma, potentially hindering individuals from seeking help for binge eating or related concerns. Addressing mental health within cultural frameworks is crucial for effective support and intervention.

Cultural Competence in Healthcare

Recognizing and respecting cultural perspectives is essential in providing healthcare sensitive to diverse backgrounds. Healthcare professionals, including those addressing binge eating, should cultivate cultural competence to understand the unique influences on individuals' relationships with food and mental health.

Conclusion

Cultural perspectives on food weave a rich tapestry, shaping how individuals perceive, engage with, and derive meaning from their meals. Recognizing the impact of cultural norms, traditions, and values on eating behaviors, including binge eating, is crucial for fostering a holistic understanding of individuals' relationships with food. By embracing cultural diversity, promoting cultural competence in healthcare, and encouraging open dialogues around cultural influences on mental health, society can contribute to a more inclusive and supportive approach to individuals navigating the complex intersection of culture and eating behaviors.

Cultural Perspectives on Eating

Eating is a cultural act deeply woven into identity, tradition, and societal norms. The lens through which different cultures approach and perceive eating is diverse and rich. This exploration delves into the multifaceted realm of cultural perspectives on eating, uncovering the traditions, values, and social dynamics that shape individuals' relationships with food within varying cultural contexts.

1. Cultural Traditions and Eating Rituals

Mealtime as Ritual

In many cultures, mealtime is more than a biological necessity; it's a tradition-based ritual. Cultural practices surrounding meal preparation, serving, and sharing are often significant, reinforcing a sense of community, family bonds, and cultural identity. These rituals contribute to a holistic understanding of eating beyond mere sustenance.

Festive Eating and Celebrations

Cultural perspectives on eating are intimately tied to celebrations and festivals. Traditional dishes prepared during cultural festivities serve not only to nourish but also to commemorate and pass down cultural heritage. However, the festive nature of these occasions may also contribute to a complex relationship with food, potentially influencing binge eating behaviors.

2. Diversity in Culinary Traditions

Regional and Ethnic Culinary Diversity

Cultural perspectives on eating manifest in the diverse culinary traditions that span regions and ethnicities. Each culture brings a unique flavor palette, ingredients, and cooking methods to the global table. Understanding and appreciating this diversity fosters cultural sensitivity and enriches individuals' culinary experiences.

Cultural Fusion and Globalization

In an era of globalization, cultural perspectives on eating evolve through fusion and cross-cultural influences. Traditional dishes may undergo reinterpretation or blending with elements from other cuisines. While this creates culinary diversity, it also introduces new challenges in navigating cultural authenticity and its impact on eating behaviors.

3. Cultural Significance of Specific Foods
Symbolic Meaning of Ingredients

Certain foods hold symbolic importance within cultural contexts. Ingredients may be imbued with meanings related to spirituality, seasons, or historical events. The cultural significance of these foods contributes to a nuanced understanding of eating practices, influencing individuals' relationships with specific ingredients and their potential role in binge eating triggers.

Food as Medicine in Traditional Practices

In some cultures, specific foods are revered for their perceived medicinal properties. Traditional healing practices often incorporate dietary guidelines that view food as a form of medicine. While this approach contributes to holistic well-being, it may also impact individuals' relationships with food, potentially influencing eating behaviors.

4. Cultural Perspectives on Portion Control

Variability in Portion Norms

Cultural perspectives on portion sizes vary widely. Some cultures prioritize moderation and portion control, emphasizing balance and satisfaction without excess. Others may celebrate abundance and generosity in portions. Understanding these cultural norms is essential for appreciating diverse attitudes toward eating and avoiding misunderstandings related to portion expectations.

Cultural Influences on Eating Pace

Eating pace, or the speed at which meals are consumed, is influenced by cultural norms. Some cultures value leisurely, communal dining experiences that stretch over extended periods. In contrast, others may prioritize efficiency and quicker meals. These cultural differences can influence individuals' relationships with eating and potentially impact binge eating patterns.

5. Social Dynamics and Communal Eating Practices

Communal Meals as Social Glue

Cultural perspectives often emphasize communal eating practices to foster social bonds. Sharing meals with family, friends, or the community is vital. However, the communal nature of dining may also introduce social pressures, potentially influencing individuals' behaviors, including emotional triggers for binge eating in social settings.

<u>Cultural Etiquette and Eating Norms</u>

Cultural norms dictate specific etiquette and behaviors during meals. Understanding and adhering to these cultural expectations is crucial for individuals navigating diverse social settings. Deviations from cultural eating norms may lead to feelings of discomfort or social pressure, potentially influencing eating behaviors.

6. Navigating Cultural Identity and Eating Disorders

<u>Cultural Identity Conflicts and Eating Behaviors</u>

For individuals navigating multiple cultural identities, conflicts may arise in terms of eating behaviors. Balancing the expectations of different cultural contexts may introduce challenges, potentially influencing the development or exacerbation of disordered eating patterns, including binge eating.

Cultural Competence in Healthcare

Healthcare providers must be culturally competent to understand the nuances of individuals' relationships with food within specific cultural contexts. Recognizing how cultural perspectives on eating intersect with mental health and eating disorders is essential for providing effective, culturally sensitive support and interventions.

Conclusion

Cultural perspectives on eating form a dynamic and diverse tapestry, profoundly shaping individuals' relationships with food. Recognizing the cultural significance of rituals, ingredients, and social dynamics is crucial for fostering cultural sensitivity and understanding the complexities of eating behaviors, including binge eating, within diverse cultural contexts. Embracing this cultural diversity contributes to a more inclusive, respectful, and supportive approach to individuals' relationships with food across the global spectrum.

Chapter 4

Biological Factors

Embark on a journey into the intricate interplay between biology and binge eating. This chapter delves into genetic influences, neurological orchestrations, and hormonal symphonies that shape our eating behaviors. From unraveling the genetic component to exploring the subtle dance of hormones regulating hunger, join us in deciphering the biological factors that contribute to the complex landscape of binge eating.

In tis chapter, we will look at

1. Genetics and Binge Eating

    ★ Understanding the Genetic Component

★ Neurological Influences on Eating Behavior

2. Hormones and Appetite

   ★ Exploring the Hormonal Regulation of Hunger

   ★ Impact on Binge Eating

Genetics and Binge Eating

Step into the realm where DNA whispers secrets about our relationship with food. In this exploration, we venture into the genetic landscape, unlocking the mysteries that may influence our propensity for binge eating. As we peer into the intricacies of our genetic code, join the quest to understand how heredity shapes our journey with food, shedding light on genetics' role in the tapestry of binge eating behaviors.

Understanding the Genetic Component

Genetics plays a pivotal role in shaping various aspects of our physical and mental traits, and the realm of binge eating is no exception. Investigating the genetic component provides insight into the potential hereditary factors contributing to binge eating behaviours' development and manifestation.

1. Genetic Predisposition and Familial Patterns

Inherited Susceptibility

Research suggests that individuals may inherit a predisposition to certain eating behaviors, including binge eating, through genetic factors. Familial patterns of disordered eating may highlight a genetic link, as individuals with a family history of binge eating disorders may be more susceptible to developing similar ways.

<u>**Genetic Variation and Risk**</u>

Specific genetic variations have been identified in studies examining binge eating behaviors. Variants related to neurotransmitter systems, appetite regulation, and reward pathways may contribute to an increased risk of binge eating tendencies, emphasizing the complex interplay between genetic factors and environmental influences.

2. Neurotransmitter Systems and Binge Eating

<u>**Dopamine and Reward Pathways**</u>

Neurotransmitters, chemical messengers in the brain, are crucial in regulating mood, appetite, and reward. Genetic variations in dopamine receptors, a key player in reward pathways, have been linked to binge eating tendencies. Understanding these genetic influences provides insights into the neurological underpinnings of compulsive eating behaviors.

Serotonin and Mood Regulation

Genetic factors related to serotonin, a neurotransmitter associated with mood regulation, may also contribute to binge eating. Variations in serotonin receptor genes have been implicated in the development of disordered eating patterns, shedding light on the connection between genetic factors and emotional aspects of binge eating.

3. Appetite Regulation Genes

Leptin and Ghrelin Dynamics

Genetic factors influence the regulation of appetite hormones, such as leptin and ghrelin. Leptin, produced by fat cells, signals feelings of fullness, while ghrelin stimulates hunger. Genetic variations in these appetite-regulating genes may impact an individual's susceptibility to binge eating by influencing hunger cues and satiety.

<u>Insulin Resistance and Metabolic Factors</u>

Genetic factors related to insulin resistance and metabolic functions may contribute to binge eating behaviors. Disruptions in insulin signaling and glucose metabolism, influenced by genetic variations, can affect energy balance and contribute to heightened cravings, potentially influencing the development of binge eating patterns.

4. Gene-Environment Interactions

<u>Epigenetics and Environmental Influences</u>

The interaction between genes and the environment, known as epigenetics, plays a crucial role in shaping behavior. Genetic predispositions may interact with environmental factors, such as stress or trauma, influencing the expression of genes related to binge eating.

Understanding these interactions provides a more nuanced view of the interplay between genetics and environmental influences.

Adaptive Evolutionary Perspectives

Some researchers propose that certain genetic predispositions to binge eating may have evolved as adaptive responses to environmental challenges. In ancestral environments where food scarcity was a threat, individuals genetically inclined to consume more during periods of abundance may have had a survival advantage. In modern contexts of food abundance, these genetic predispositions may contribute to maladaptive eating patterns.

5. Implications for Treatment and Prevention

Personalized Approaches to Intervention

Understanding the genetic component of binge eating has implications for personalized treatment approaches. Recognizing individual genetic profiles may inform therapeutic strategies, allowing for more targeted interventions tailored to an individual's genetic predispositions and neurobiological factors.

<u>Preventive Strategies Based on Genetic Risk</u>

Genetic insights also open avenues for preventive strategies. Identifying individuals at a higher genetic risk for binge eating may enable early interventions, including behavioral and psychological approaches, to mitigate the development of disordered eating patterns.

<u>Conclusion</u>

As we unravel the genetic component of binge eating, it becomes evident that our DNA holds valuable clues to the complexities of this behavior. Genetic predispositions, neurotransmitter dynamics, and appetite regulation genes collectively contribute to the intricate tapestry of binge eating. Acknowledging these genetic factors enhances our understanding of the origins of binge eating. It paves the way for more targeted and personalized approaches to prevention and treatment.

Neurological Influences on Eating Behavior

The intricate dance of neurotransmitters and neural circuits within the brain orchestrates our eating behaviors, shaping the delicate balance between hunger, satiety, and reward. In the realm of binge eating, neurological influences play a significant role in unraveling the mysteries of compulsive and dysregulated eating patterns.

1. Dopamine and the Reward Pathway
Reward-Seeking Behavior

Dopamine, a neurotransmitter associated with pleasure and reward, is central to the brain's reward pathway. Genetic and neurological factors influence the regulation of dopamine, impacting an individual's predisposition to seek rewarding experiences, including those related to food. Dysregulation of this system may contribute to the development of binge eating behaviors.

<u>Impulsivity and Dopaminergic Dynamics</u>

Dopamine's influence extends to impulsivity, a trait associated with the inability to resist immediate gratification. Neurological variations in dopamine receptor activity may contribute to heightened impulsivity, potentially influencing binge eating as individuals succumb to the immediate pleasure derived from consuming large quantities of food.

2. Serotonin and Mood Regulation

Role in Emotional Well-Being

Serotonin, another neurotransmitter, is intricately linked to mood regulation and emotional well-being. Neurological factors affecting serotonin levels may influence an individual's susceptibility to mood disorders, contributing to emotional triggers for binge eating. Variations in serotonin receptors play a role in the emotional aspects of compulsive eating behaviors.

Stress Response and Neurotransmitter Dynamics

Neurological influences on eating behaviors are heightened during stress. Chronic stress can lead to dysregulation of neurotransmitters, particularly serotonin, impacting mood and the ability to cope with emotional distress. Binge eating may emerge as a maladaptive coping mechanism in response to altered neurological responses to stress.

3. Hypothalamus and Appetite Regulation

Central Control of Hunger and Satiety

The hypothalamus, a key brain region, is the central control center for appetite regulation—neurons in the hypothalamus sense hormonal signals related to hunger and satiety. Neurological factors influencing hypothalamic function may disrupt the delicate balance, contributing to an altered perception of hunger and satiety, potentially leading to binge eating.

Leptin and Ghrelin Signaling

Neurological circuits in the hypothalamus respond to hormones such as leptin and ghrelin, which signal the body's energy status. Variations in neurological pathways involved in leptin and ghrelin signaling may impact an individual's ability to regulate appetite, contributing to overconsumption and binge eating episodes.

4. Frontal Cortex and Executive Functions

Executive Functions and Inhibitory Control

The frontal cortex, responsible for executive functions such as decision-making and inhibitory control, is crucial in regulating eating behaviors. Neurological factors influencing the frontal cortex may compromise inhibitory control, leading to impulsive and compulsive eating behaviors characteristic of binge eating.

Cognitive Flexibility and Adaptability

The frontal cortex also governs cognitive flexibility, adapting to changing situations. Neurological variations affecting cognitive flexibility may contribute to rigid eating patterns, making it challenging for individuals with binge eating tendencies to adopt healthier eating behaviors in response to changing circumstances.

5. Neurotransmitter Imbalances and Eating Disorders

Imbalances in GABA and Glutamate

The balance between inhibitory neurotransmitters like gamma-aminobutyric acid (GABA) and excitatory neurotransmitters like glutamate is crucial for neurological function. Imbalances in these neurotransmitter systems have been implicated in eating disorders, including binge eating. Neurological factors that disrupt this balance may contribute to dysregulated eating behaviors.

Neuroplasticity and Habit Formation

Neuroplasticity, the brain's ability to reorganize itself, plays a role in habit formation. Neurological factors influencing plasticity may contribute to developing and reinforcing habits associated with binge eating. Understanding these processes sheds light on the neurological mechanisms that sustain compulsive eating behaviors.

6. Therapeutic Implications and Interventions

<u>Neuroscience-Informed Therapies</u>

Advancements in neuroscience inform therapeutic interventions for binge eating. Cognitive-behavioural therapies and mindfulness-based approaches leverage our understanding of neurological influences to address maladaptive thought patterns and enhance self-regulation, offering individuals effective tools to manage and prevent binge eating episodes.

<u>Pharmacological Approaches</u>

Pharmacological interventions target neurological pathways involved in appetite regulation and reward systems. Medications that modulate neurotransmitter activity may be prescribed in conjunction with psychotherapy to address the neurological underpinnings of binge eating, providing a comprehensive approach to treatment.

Conclusion

Neurological influences intricately shape our eating behaviors, and understanding the brain's role is paramount in the context of binge eating. From the intricate dance of dopamine in reward pathways to the delicate balance in the hypothalamus regulating hunger and satiety, neurological factors paint a detailed portrait of the mechanisms underlying compulsive eating behaviors. This exploration enhances our comprehension of binge eating. It opens avenues for targeted interventions informed by the intricate workings of the brain.

Hormones and Appetite

Enter the realm where hormones orchestrate the intricate dance of appetite regulation. This exploration unravels the endocrine symphony that influences hunger cues, satiety signals, and the delicate balance between nourishment and indulgence. Join us as we delve into the hormonal realm, shedding light on how these biochemical messengers shape our relationship with food, with a particular focus on their impact on binge eating behaviors.

Exploring the Hormonal Regulation of Hunger: Unraveling the Endocrine Tapestry

Hunger, a primal sensation, is intricately woven into the fabric of our physiological experience, governed by a symphony of hormones orchestrating the complex dance between appetite and satiety. This exploration delves into the hormonal regulation of hunger, shedding light on the endocrine players that signal the body's need for sustenance and contribute to the nuanced landscape of eating behaviors.

1. Ghrelin: The Hunger Hormone

Origins and Release Dynamics

Ghrelin, often called the "hunger hormone," originates primarily in the stomach and is released in response to an empty stomach. Its levels rise before meals, signalling the brain that it's time to eat. Understanding the dynamics of ghrelin release provides insights into the initial stages of hunger and the initiation of the eating process.

Role in Appetite Stimulation

Ghrelin's primary role is to stimulate appetite. It acts on the hypothalamus, triggering the release of neuropeptides that promote hunger and enhance the rewarding aspects of food consumption. Variations in ghrelin levels may influence an individual's susceptibility to intense hunger and, consequently, their potential vulnerability to binge eating behaviors.

2. Leptin: The Satiety Signal

Produced by Adipose Tissue

Leptin is a key satiety signal produced primarily by adipose (fat) tissue. As fat stores increase, leptin levels rise, sending signals to the brain that the body has sufficient energy reserves. Understanding leptin's role provides insights into the mechanisms contributing to feelings of fullness and regulating energy balance.

Impact on Appetite Suppression

Leptin acts on the hypothalamus to suppress appetite and increase energy expenditure. Individuals with leptin deficiencies or resistance may experience reduced satiety signals, potentially leading to overeating and a heightened susceptibility to binge eating. Unraveling the intricacies of leptin's actions provides crucial insights into appetite regulation.

3. Insulin: Balancing Blood Sugar and Hunger

Regulation of Glucose Levels

While primarily known for its role in glucose regulation, insulin also influences hunger. Insulin is released in response to food consumption, facilitating glucose uptake into cells. The interplay between insulin and hunger involves regulating blood sugar levels, with fluctuations potentially influencing feelings of hunger or satiety.

Hormonal Interactions with Ghrelin and Leptin

Insulin's interactions with ghrelin and leptin contribute to the delicate balance of hunger and satiety. Dysregulation in insulin sensitivity may disrupt this balance, potentially influencing eating behaviors. Understanding the interconnected hormonal pathways provides a comprehensive view of the endocrine regulation of appetite.

4. Peptide YY (PYY) and Cholecystokinin (CCK): Satiety Peptides

Released Post-Meal

Peptide YY (PYY) and cholecystokinin (CCK) are released in response to food intake, particularly fats and proteins. These satiety peptides contribute to the feelings of fullness and satisfaction that follow a meal. Exploring the dynamics of PYY and CCK release offers insights into the post-meal satiety mechanisms that influence eating patterns.

Interactions with the Gut-Brain Axis

PYY and CCK interact with the gut-brain axis, communicating signals between the digestive system and the brain to regulate appetite. Dysfunction in this axis may contribute to disruptions in the satiety signaling process, potentially influencing an individual's vulnerability to overeating and binge eating.

5. Peptide Hormones and the Gut-Brain Axis

Integration of Signals

The gut-brain axis integrates signals from various peptide hormones, neurotransmitters, and sensory inputs to regulate appetite. Understanding how these signals are processed and integrated within the brain provides a holistic perspective on the complexities of appetite regulation and the intricate mechanisms that contribute to binge eating tendencies.

Neurological Modulation of Hormonal Signals

Neurological factors are crucial in modulating hormonal signals related to hunger and satiety. Neurotransmitters, neural circuits, and brain regions involved in appetite regulation interact with hormonal pathways to fine-tune the delicate balance between eating initiation and termination.

Conclusion

Exploring the hormonal regulation of hunger unveils the intricate tapestry of biochemical messengers orchestrating our appetite and satiety. From the ghrelin-driven initiation of hunger to the leptin-mediated fullness signals, these hormones create a dynamic interplay that shapes our relationship with food. Understanding these endocrine intricacies enhances our comprehension of appetite regulation. It provides valuable insights into the hormonal factors contributing to binge eating behaviors.

Impact on Binge Eating

The intricate interplay of hormones in the endocrine system extends its influence beyond mere physiological processes, delving into the complex realm of appetite regulation and its potential impact on binge eating behaviors. Understanding how hormonal dynamics contribute to the vulnerability and manifestation of binge eating sheds light on the nuanced connections between biochemistry and compulsive eating patterns.

1. Ghrelin's Role in Binge Eating Vulnerability

Heightened Appetite Stimulation

As the instigator of hunger, Ghrelin plays a critical role in binge eating vulnerability. Individuals with higher baseline ghrelin levels or heightened sensitivity to ghrelin may experience more intense feelings of hunger, potentially driving them towards larger and more frequent meals, a behavioral pattern linked to binge eating tendencies.

<u>Emotional Triggers and Ghrelin Response</u>

The relationship between ghrelin and emotional triggers further complicates the landscape. Stress and emotional distress can lead to an increase in ghrelin levels, creating a biochemical environment that amplifies the susceptibility to emotional eating, a precursor to binge eating episodes.

2. Leptin Resistance and Dysregulated Satiety Signals

<u>Reduced Responsiveness to Fullness</u>

Leptin resistance, a condition where the body's cells become less responsive to leptin signals, contributes to dysregulated satiety signals. Individuals with leptin resistance may experience reduced sensations of fullness, potentially leading to overeating and the continuation of eating beyond physiological needs, a hallmark of binge eating behaviors.

Role in Reward-Based Eating

Leptin's involvement in the brain's reward pathways adds a layer of complexity. Dysregulation in leptin signaling may contribute to a reduced sensitivity to the rewarding aspects of food consumption, driving individuals with binge eating tendencies to seek heightened reward through larger and more calorically dense meals.

3. Insulin Resistance and the Craving Cycle

Impact on Cravings and Appetite

Insulin resistance, commonly associated with metabolic disorders, can impact appetite regulation. Elevated insulin levels may increase cravings for carbohydrates, particularly sugary and processed foods. The cyclic nature of insulin resistance and cravings creates a scenario conducive to binge eating, as individuals succumb to the urge to consume highly palatable foods.

Energy Imbalance and Compulsive Eating

Insulin resistance may disrupt the delicate balance between energy intake and expenditure. This imbalance, coupled with heightened cravings, can result in periods of overconsumption and subsequent compensatory behaviors, contributing to a pattern of the compulsive eating characteristic of binge eating episodes.

4. Peptide YY (PYY) and Cholecystokinin (CCK) in Post-Meal Satisfaction

<u>Delayed Satiety Signals</u>

In individuals prone to binge eating, delayed or blunted satiety signals mediated by PYY and CCK may play a role. Reduced sensitivity to these post-meal satiety peptides can result in a shortened duration of feelings of fullness, potentially leading to a faster return to a state of hunger and increasing the likelihood of overeating.

<u>Gut-Brain Axis Dysfunction</u>

Dysfunction in the gut-brain axis, which involves the interplay between gastrointestinal hormones and neural signals, may contribute to an impaired response to satiety cues. Individuals with disrupted gut-brain communication may struggle to regulate their food intake effectively, fostering an environment conducive to binge eating.

5. Interactions with Psychological and Environmental Factors

<u>Psychological Impact of Hormonal Dysregulation</u>

The impact of hormonal dysregulation extends beyond the physiological realm, influencing psychological aspects of binge eating. Hormonal imbalances can contribute to mood swings, increased stress, and emotional reactivity, further intertwining biological and psychological factors that drive maladaptive eating behaviors.

<u>Environmental Triggers and Hormonal Response</u>

Environmental factors, such as the availability of highly palatable foods and societal pressures, interact with hormonal dynamics. Food cues and societal norms may amplify hormonal responses to appetite-related signals, creating an environment where hormonal imbalances align with external triggers to promote binge-eating behaviors.

Conclusion

The impact of hormonal dynamics on binge eating is a multifaceted exploration of biochemical intricacies and their interconnectedness with psychological and environmental factors. Ghrelin's role in hunger initiation, leptin's influence on satiety, insulin's impact on cravings, and the post-meal satisfaction signals of PYY and CCK collectively shape the landscape of compulsive eating behaviors. Recognizing the interplay between hormones and binge eating provides a comprehensive perspective for interventions targeting both the physiological and psychological aspects of this complex eating disorder.

Chapter 5

Breaking the Stigma

In a world often clouded by misconceptions, this chapter seeks to unravel the truths concealed behind the stigma of binge eating. By dispelling myths, challenging stereotypes, and fostering understanding, we embark on a journey to promote compassion. It's time to rewrite the narrative, replacing judgment with empathy and unveiling the complexities surrounding binge eating.

In this chapter, we are going to look at

1. Dispelling Myths about Binge Eating

    ★ Challenging Stereotypes

    ★ Promoting Understanding and Compassion

Dispelling Myths about Binge Eating

In the realm of binge eating, myths abound, casting shadows on the realities of this complex and often misunderstood disorder. This section is dedicated to illuminating the truths obscured by misconceptions. By dismantling myths, we pave the way for a more precise understanding, fostering empathy and a path towards effective support and recovery. Let's embark on a journey to unravel the reality behind the myths that shroud binge eating in misinformation.

Challenging Stereotypes

Stereotypes surrounding binge eating perpetuate misunderstandings and hinder genuine empathy. In this exploration, we challenge these stereotypes, seeking to replace judgment with a compassionate understanding of the complexities underlying binge eating. By debunking misconceptions, we aim to foster a more inclusive and supportive approach to individuals navigating the challenges of this disorder.

1. Myth: Binge Eating is a Lack of Willpower

Reality: A Complex Behavioral Disorder

Binge eating is not a simple manifestation of weak willpower. It is a complex behavioral disorder with roots in psychological, biological, and environmental factors. Individuals grappling with binge eating often face challenges beyond mere self-control, and understanding this complexity is crucial for dismantling the stereotype that frames it as a choice rather than a disorder.

2. Myth: Only Overweight Individuals Struggle with Binge Eating

<u>**Reality:** Binge Eating Affects Individuals of All Body Types</u>

Contrary to the stereotype linking binge eating exclusively to overweight individuals, this disorder does not discriminate based on body size. Individuals with binge eating disorder may present with various body types, challenging the assumption that one's weight is a reliable indicator of their relationship with food. Challenging this stereotype is vital for recognizing and addressing binge eating across diverse populations.

3. Myth: Binge Eating is Simply Overeating

<u>**Reality:** Distinct Characteristics of Binge Eating Disorder</u>

Binge eating is not synonymous with occasional overeating. It is characterized by recurrent episodes of consuming large quantities of food, accompanied by a sense of loss of control. Understanding the distinct features of binge eating disorder is essential for dispelling the myth that lumps it together with common overindulgence, recognizing it as a clinically significant mental health condition.

4. Myth: Binge Eating is Always Visible

Reality: Hidden Struggles and Shame

The stereotype that binge eating is always observable overlooks the hidden struggles individuals may face. Many people with binge eating disorder suffer in silence, consumed by shame and guilt. Challenging the notion that binge eating is always visible is crucial for acknowledging individuals' internal battles and creating a space for open dialogue and support.

5. Myth: Binge Eating is a Choice or Attention-Seeking Behavior

Reality: <u>A Coping Mechanism for Underlying Issues</u>

Binge eating is not a conscious choice or a bid for attention. It often serves as a coping mechanism for underlying emotional, psychological, or environmental stressors. Dispelling the myth that frames binge eating as attention-seeking allows for a more empathetic understanding of the deeper issues individuals may be grappling with.

6. Myth: Binge Eating is Easy to Overcome with Willpower Alone

Reality: <u>Requires Comprehensive Treatment and Support</u>

Overcoming binge eating is not a straightforward task of willpower. It necessitates a comprehensive approach, including psychological therapy, nutritional guidance, and support networks. Challenging the stereotype that individuals can conquer binge eating through sheer willpower alone underscores the importance of recognizing the multifaceted nature of this disorder.

Conclusion

Challenging stereotypes surrounding binge eating is a crucial step toward fostering a compassionate and informed perspective. By dismantling misconceptions, we pave the way for a more supportive environment that recognizes the complexities of this disorder. This shift in perception is integral to promoting understanding, reducing stigma, and providing meaningful support to individuals on their journey toward recovery from binge eating disorder.

Promoting Understanding and Compassion

To foster empathy and dispel stigma, this section is dedicated to promoting understanding and compassion for individuals navigating binge eating challenges. By unraveling the complexities of this disorder, we aim to build bridges of support and awareness, fostering a more compassionate society that recognizes the humanity behind the struggle.

1. Understanding the Complexity of Binge Eating

Holistic Perspective on Binge Eating Disorder

To promote understanding, it's crucial to embrace a holistic perspective on binge eating disorder. Recognizing the intricate interplay of biological, psychological, and environmental factors helps dispel the notion that this disorder is a simple matter of willpower. Understanding the complexity opens the door to empathy and allows for more effective support and intervention.

2. The Role of Mental Health in Binge Eating

Acknowledging Mental Health Impacts

Binge eating is deeply intertwined with mental health, often serving as a coping mechanism for emotional distress. By acknowledging the mental health impacts, we promote a compassionate approach that views binge eating as a symptom rather than a character flaw. Encouraging open conversations about mental health reduces stigma and encourages seeking professional help.

3. Breaking Down Barriers to Seeking Help

Reducing Stigma around Treatment

Promoting understanding involves breaking down barriers to seeking help. Many individuals with binge eating disorders face internalized stigma that hinders their willingness to reach out for support. By fostering an environment that normalizes seeking help and emphasizing the effectiveness of evidence-based treatments, we encourage individuals to take the crucial step towards recovery.

4. Educating Communities on Binge Eating Disorder

<u>Community Awareness Programs</u>

Promoting compassion requires a broader understanding within communities. Education programs that raise awareness about binge eating disorder can help dispel myths and foster empathy. By reaching schools, workplaces, and community organizations, we create a culture of understanding that supports individuals dealing with binge eating and contributes to reducing societal stigma.

5. Encouraging Empathy in Support Networks

Family and Friend Support

For those with binge eating disorder, support networks play a pivotal role. Encouraging empathy within these circles involves educating family and friends about the nature of the disorder. Emphasizing the role of compassion in offering support rather than judgment creates an environment where individuals feel understood and accepted on their journey to recovery.

6. Media Representation and Destigmatization

Responsible Portrayal in Media

Media has a powerful influence on public perception. Promoting understanding involves advocating for responsible and accurate portrayals of binge eating disorders in media. By destigmatizing the disorder through realistic depictions and informed narratives, we contribute to a culture that fosters empathy and rejects harmful stereotypes.

7. Incorporating Compassion into Treatment Approaches

Therapeutic Compassion Practices

In treatment settings, incorporating compassion-focused approaches enhances the healing process. Therapeutic practices that emphasize self-compassion and understanding reduce feelings of shame and guilt. By addressing the emotional aspects of binge eating, treatment becomes more holistic and supportive, promoting lasting recovery.

Conclusion

Promoting understanding and compassion for individuals grappling with binge eating disorder is a collective responsibility. By embracing the complexities of this condition, breaking down barriers to seeking help, and fostering empathy within communities, we create a society that supports rather than stigmatizes. This compassionate approach not only aids those directly affected but contributes to a broader culture of empathy and awareness surrounding mental health challenges.

Chapter 6

Seeking Professional Help

Embarking on the journey toward recovery from binge eating requires professional guidance and support. This chapter explores therapeutic approaches and medical interventions that form the foundation of comprehensive treatment. From the cognitive restructuring of Cognitive-Behavioral Therapy (CBT) to the dialectical insights of Dialectical Behavior Therapy (DBT), we delve into the various avenues individuals can explore. Additionally, we unravel the role of medications and the crucial support healthcare professionals provide on the path to healing. Let's navigate the diverse landscape of seeking professional help for overcoming binge eating.

In this chapter, you are going to learn:

1. Therapeutic Approaches

    ★ Cognitive-Behavioral Therapy (CBT)

    ★ Dialectical Behavior Therapy (DBT)

    ★ Interpersonal Psychotherapy (IPT)

2. Medical Interventions

    ★ Medications and Binge Eating

    ★ The Role of Healthcare Professionals

Therapeutic Approaches

Within the realm of overcoming binge eating, therapeutic approaches stand as beacons of hope and guidance. This section illuminates the diverse methodologies individuals can explore on their journey to recovery. From the cognitive restructuring of Cognitive-Behavioral Therapy (CBT) to the interpersonal insights of Interpersonal Psychotherapy (IPT) and the dialectical strategies of Dialectical Behavior Therapy (DBT), we embark on a comprehensive exploration of the therapeutic avenues that pave the way for lasting healing.

Cognitive-Behavioral Therapy (CBT) for Binge Eating

Cognitive-Behavioral Therapy (CBT) stands as a cornerstone in the therapeutic landscape for binge eating, offering a structured and evidence-based approach to address the intertwined cognitive and behavioral aspects of this disorder. By targeting distorted thought patterns, fostering self-awareness, and instigating behavioral change, CBT provides individuals with practical tools to break free from the cycle of binge eating.

1. Understanding the Core Principles of CBT

Cognitive Restructuring

At the heart of CBT lies cognitive restructuring, which involves identifying and challenging distorted thoughts related to food, body image, and self-worth. By recognizing and reframing these negative cognitions, individuals can cultivate a healthier mindset, reducing the triggers that lead to binge eating episodes.

Behavioral Activation

CBT incorporates behavioral activation to encourage individuals to engage in positive activities and establish healthier routines. By fostering constructive behaviors, individuals can disrupt the patterns of isolation and sedentary habits often associated with binge eating, promoting a more balanced and fulfilling lifestyle.

2. Identifying Triggers and Developing Coping Strategies

Trigger Analysis

CBT guides individuals in identifying the specific triggers that precede binge eating episodes. Whether rooted in emotions, stressors, or environmental cues, understanding these triggers is pivotal. This process allows for targeted interventions to address the underlying issues contributing to binge eating.

Coping Skills Development

Once triggers are identified, CBT equips individuals with a toolbox of coping skills. These skills encompass healthier ways of managing stress, emotional distress, and challenging situations without binge eating. Learning and implementing effective coping strategies empower individuals to navigate life's challenges more adaptively.

3. Establishing and Monitoring Goals

Setting Realistic Objectives

CBT involves collaboratively setting realistic and achievable goals with the individual. These goals relate to improving eating patterns, addressing emotional well-being, or establishing a more positive relationship with food. The step-by-step approach ensures that individuals progress at a pace aligned with their capabilities and readiness for change.

Monitoring Progress and Adjusting Strategies

Regularly monitoring progress is a crucial component of CBT. This involves assessing the effectiveness of strategies, identifying areas that require adjustment, and celebrating successes.

The iterative nature of this process ensures that therapeutic interventions remain tailored to the individual's evolving needs.

4. Mindfulness and CBT Integration

Enhancing Self-Awareness through Mindfulness

CBT often integrates mindfulness practices to enhance self-awareness. Mindfulness encourages individuals to observe their thoughts and feelings without judgment, fostering a non-reactive awareness of the present moment. This heightened self-awareness aligns with CBT principles, enabling individuals to disentangle themselves from automatic, negative thought patterns.

Mindful Eating Practices

CBT incorporates mindful eating practices to reshape individuals' relationships with food. Individuals develop a more attuned and balanced approach to meals by promoting awareness of hunger and fullness cues and the sensory aspects of eating. Mindful eating aligns with CBT's goals of disrupting automatic and impulsive eating behaviors.

5. Group and Individual Formats of CBT

Group Therapy Dynamics

CBT can be delivered in both group and individual formats. Group therapy fosters a sense of community and shared experiences, providing individuals with support and understanding from peers facing similar challenges. Group settings offer a platform for exchanging coping strategies, building interpersonal skills, and reducing feelings of isolation.

Individualized Attention in One-on-One Therapy

Individual CBT sessions allow a more personalized exploration of an individual's unique experiences and challenges. The therapist tailors interventions to the specific needs and goals of the individual, providing a focused and individualized approach to addressing binge eating behaviors.

6. Long-Term Maintenance and Relapse Prevention

Building Sustainable Habits

CBT is about immediate change and focuses on building sustainable habits for long-term recovery. By instilling adaptive thought patterns and reinforcing positive behaviors, CBT equips individuals with the skills to navigate challenges independently and maintain progress beyond formal therapeutic intervention.

Relapse Prevention Strategies

Recognizing that setbacks may occur, CBT includes relapse prevention strategies. Individuals learn to identify early warning signs of potential relapse and implement coping strategies to prevent a return to unhealthy patterns. This proactive approach empowers individuals to stay resilient in facing future challenges.

Conclusion

Cognitive-Behavioral Therapy (CBT) stands as a dynamic and effective therapeutic approach for individuals grappling with binge eating. By addressing distorted thought patterns, cultivating coping skills, and promoting behavior change, CBT empowers individuals to rewrite their relationship with food and establish a foundation for lasting recovery. The integration of mindfulness, goal setting, and personalized attention makes CBT a versatile and invaluable tool in the journey toward healing from binge eating disorder.

Dialectical Behavior Therapy (DBT)

Dialectical Behavior Therapy (DBT) emerges as a transformative approach for individuals grappling with binge eating, offering a comprehensive framework that harmonizes acceptance and change. Rooted in mindfulness, emotional regulation, interpersonal effectiveness, and distress tolerance principles, DBT provides a structured path toward breaking the cycle of binge eating behaviors and fostering lasting emotional well-being.

1. **Foundations of Dialectical Behavior Therapy (DBT)**

<u>Dialectics: Balancing Opposing Concepts</u>

At the core of DBT is dialectics, encouraging individuals to find a synthesis between opposing ideas. Binge eating involves balancing acceptance of current circumstances with the commitment to change. Recognizing that ambivalence and conflicting feelings are natural, DBT helps individuals navigate these tensions to facilitate sustainable transformation.

Mindfulness as a Cornerstone

Mindfulness is a cornerstone of DBT, encouraging individuals to cultivate non-judgmental awareness of their thoughts, emotions, and behaviors. Individuals can disrupt automatic response patterns by being present at the moment, fostering a deeper understanding of the triggers and motivations underlying binge eating.

2. Emotion Regulation Skills

Identifying and Labeling Emotions

DBT equips individuals with the skills to identify and label emotions accurately. This process is crucial for understanding the emotional landscape often preceding binge eating episodes. Individuals can develop targeted strategies to regulate intense emotions effectively by enhancing emotional awareness.

Developing Healthy Coping Mechanisms

Incorporating emotion regulation skills involves developing healthy coping mechanisms. DBT provides individuals with a repertoire of strategies to manage and cope with distressing emotions without resorting to maladaptive behaviors like binge eating. This shift towards healthier coping mechanisms is integral to the long-term success of DBT.

3. Interpersonal Effectiveness Training

Assertiveness and Boundary Setting

DBT emphasizes interpersonal effectiveness, empowering individuals to navigate relationships assertively and set healthy boundaries. Building these skills is instrumental in reducing interpersonal stressors that may contribute to binge eating. Through effective communication and boundary setting, individuals enhance their ability to meet emotional needs without turning to destructive eating patterns.

<u>Building and Maintaining Relationships</u>

Interpersonal effectiveness training in DBT extends to building and maintaining relationships. Individuals learn valuable skills to connect with others authentically, fostering a sense of support and connection. Strong interpersonal relationships provide a buffer against isolation and loneliness, factors that may contribute to binge eating tendencies.

4. Distress Tolerance Techniques

<u>Crisis Survival Strategies</u>

DBT integrates distress tolerance techniques to help individuals navigate moments of crisis without resorting to harmful behaviors. These crisis survival strategies are essential for preventing impulsive actions, such as binge eating, during times of heightened emotional distress. By fostering distress tolerance, individuals build resilience and adaptive coping mechanisms.

Acceptance of Unchangeable Realities

Distress tolerance in DBT involves accepting unchangeable realities. This acknowledgment is crucial for reducing the emotional intensity of situations beyond an individual's control. By embracing acceptance, individuals minimize the emotional triggers that may lead to binge eating as a coping mechanism.

5. Individual and Group Therapy Components

Individual DBT Sessions

DBT is often delivered through a combination of individual and group therapy. Individual sessions provide a personalized exploration of an individual's experiences and challenges. Therapists tailor interventions to the individual's unique needs, fostering a collaborative and supportive therapeutic relationship.

Group Dynamics and Skills Training

Group therapy sessions in DBT serve as skills training and peer support platforms. Participants learn from one another's experiences, share coping strategies, and collectively work towards mastering the skills taught in the program. The group format enhances a sense of community and reduces feelings of isolation.

6. Application of DBT Skills to Binge Eating

Mindful Eating Practices

DBT encourages the application of mindfulness to eating behaviors. Mindful eating practices involve:

- Being fully present during meals.

- Savoring each bite.

- Paying attention to hunger and fullness cues.

This mindful approach disrupts automatic and impulsive eating patterns, fostering a healthier relationship with food.

Using Emotion Regulation in Response to Triggers

DBT skills, particularly those related to emotion regulation, are applied proactively in response to triggers for binge eating. Individuals learn to identify emotional triggers, use coping strategies to regulate intense emotions and disrupt the cycle of turning to food as a maladaptive coping mechanism.

7. Long-Term Maintenance and Integration into Daily Life

Generalization of Skills to Daily Life

DBT emphasizes the generalization of skills to daily life beyond the therapeutic setting. Individuals are encouraged to integrate learned skills into various aspects of their lives, including relationships, work, and self-care. This integration ensures that the benefits of DBT extend into long-term maintenance and sustained recovery.

Continued Support and Skill Refinement

DBT acknowledges the ongoing nature of skill refinement and support. Individuals may continue to receive support as needed, and the skill refinement process continues throughout the recovery journey. This adaptive and continuous approach aligns with the principles of DBT, fostering resilience and flexibility in the face of life's challenges.

Conclusion

Dialectical Behavior Therapy (DBT) stands as a powerful and holistic approach to addressing binge eating, blending acceptance and change within a structured framework. By fostering mindfulness, emotion regulation, interpersonal effectiveness, and distress tolerance, DBT equips individuals with a versatile toolkit for navigating life's challenges and breaking free from the cycle of binge eating. The synthesis of opposing concepts, the emphasis on mindfulness, and the incorporation of practical skills make DBT an invaluable therapeutic approach for those seeking lasting recovery from binge eating disorder.

Interpersonal Psychotherapy (IPT)

Interpersonal Psychotherapy (IPT) emerges as a compassionate and relationship-focused approach to addressing binge eating, placing interpersonal relationships at the forefront of the therapeutic process. Rooted in the belief that relationships significantly impact emotional well-being, IPT explores and navigates the interpersonal dynamics that may contribute to binge eating behaviors. By fostering self-awareness, enhancing communication skills, and addressing relational challenges, IPT offers individuals a pathway to healing from binge eating within the context of their interpersonal lives.

1. Understanding the Core Principles of Interpersonal Psychotherapy (IPT)

Interpersonal Relationships as a Catalyst for Change

IPT is founded on the principle that the quality of interpersonal relationships profoundly influences emotional health. This therapeutic approach acknowledges the impact of relationships on an individual's well-being. It explores how improving these connections can lead to a reduction in binge eating behaviors.

Time-Limited and Goal-Oriented

IPT is typically time-limited and goal-oriented, focusing on specific interpersonal issues related to binge eating. The structured nature of IPT helps individuals identify and address challenges within a defined timeframe, making it a practical and effective approach for those seeking targeted therapeutic interventions.

2. Exploration of Interpersonal Difficulties Linked to Binge Eating

Role Transitions

IPT delves into life changes and role transitions that may contribute to binge eating. These transitions, such as job changes, relationship shifts, or life-stage adjustments, can trigger emotional distress. Exploring how these transitions impact an individual's relationships and coping mechanisms is integral to the IPT process.

Grief and Loss

The experience of grief and loss is often intertwined with binge eating. IPT helps individuals navigate the emotions associated with loss and examines how these emotions may manifest in relationships. By addressing unresolved grief, individuals can develop healthier coping strategies and reduce the likelihood of turning to binge eating for emotional relief.

3. Enhancing Communication Skills and Emotional Expression

Improving Communication

IPT emphasizes enhancing communication skills to foster more effective and open interpersonal interactions. Individuals learn to express their needs, emotions, and boundaries constructively.

Improved communication reduces misunderstandings and provides a foundation for healthier relationships, diminishing the emotional triggers that lead to binge eating.

Emotional Expression within Relationships

The therapy explores how emotions are expressed within relationships, recognizing the impact of unspoken feelings on emotional well-being. IPT facilitates an environment where individuals feel safe to say and process emotions, leading to a more authentic connection with others. This emotional expression helps prevent the buildup of emotional distress that may contribute to binge eating.

4. Identifying Patterns in Relationships and Binge Eating Behaviors

Role of Relationships in Binge Eating

IPT examines the patterns within relationships that may contribute to binge eating behaviors. It explores how interpersonal conflicts, unmet emotional needs, or dysfunctional relationship dynamics may serve as triggers for maladaptive eating patterns. Identifying these patterns is crucial for developing targeted interventions to break the cycle.

Attachment Styles and Binge Eating

Attachment styles, rooted in early relationships, are explored within IPT. Understanding how attachment patterns influence current relationships and coping mechanisms provides valuable insights. By addressing insecure attachment styles and fostering secure connections, individuals can reduce reliance on binge eating as a means of emotional regulation.

5. Strategies for Resolving Interpersonal Conflicts

Conflict Resolution Techniques

IPT equips individuals with practical strategies for resolving interpersonal conflicts. By developing conflict resolution skills, individuals can navigate relationship challenges more effectively, reducing the emotional distress that may contribute to binge eating. Improved conflict resolution promotes a healthier emotional environment.

<u>Negotiating Expectations and Boundaries</u>

Negotiating expectations and setting healthy boundaries are crucial components of IPT. Individuals learn to establish clear expectations within relationships and set boundaries that promote emotional well-being. Clear communication and boundary-setting contribute to a more stable interpersonal foundation, reducing the likelihood of turning to binge eating.

6. Improving Self-Esteem and Self-Perception

<u>Self-Esteem and Relationship Dynamics</u>

IPT addresses the interplay between self-esteem and interpersonal relationships. Exploring how self-perception influences relationship dynamics provides a framework for building a more positive self-image. Improved self-esteem contributes to emotional resilience and reduces vulnerability to binge eating as a coping mechanism.

<u>Promoting Self-Compassion within Relationships</u>

IPT encourages the cultivation of self-compassion within the context of relationships. Individuals learn to approach themselves with kindness and understanding, fostering a more nurturing internal dialogue. By promoting self-compassion, IPT reduces the emotional turmoil that may lead to binge eating.

7. Integration of Interpersonal Insights into Daily Life

Applying IPT Insights to Relationships

IPT emphasizes the application of insights gained in therapy to real-life relationships. Individuals are encouraged to implement the communication skills, conflict resolution strategies, and emotional expression techniques learned in therapy into their daily interactions. This integration supports the generalization of therapeutic gains beyond the therapeutic setting.

Building a Supportive Social Network

As part of IPT, individuals are encouraged to build a supportive social network. Strengthening connections with friends and family provides additional support and reduces feelings of isolation. A robust social network contributes to emotional resilience and diminishes the reliance on binge eating for emotional relief.

Conclusion

Interpersonal Psychotherapy (IPT) stands as a relational and goal-oriented approach for individuals seeking to overcome binge eating. By exploring the impact of interpersonal dynamics on emotional well-being, improving communication skills, and addressing relationship patterns, IPT offers a nuanced pathway to healing. The integration of insights into daily life and the emphasis on fostering supportive connections make IPT a valuable therapeutic approach for those striving towards lasting recovery from binge eating disorder.

Medical Interventions

In the multifaceted journey to address binge eating, medical interventions serve as a vital bridge between science and personalized support. This section delves into the pharmacological and healthcare dimensions of recovery, exploring how medications can play a role in managing binge eating disorder. Additionally, we unravel the indispensable contributions of healthcare professionals in providing holistic care, ensuring individuals receive comprehensive support on their path to healing. Let's explore the intersection of medical science and compassionate care in the pursuit of overcoming binge eating.

Medications and Binge Eating

Medical interventions, specifically medications, form a distinctive facet in the comprehensive approach to addressing binge eating disorder. While therapeutic modalities like psychotherapy play a crucial role, certain medications have shown efficacy in managing symptoms and promoting recovery. In this exploration, we delve into the pharmacological landscape of medications used to treat binge eating, understanding their mechanisms, benefits, and considerations within the broader context of holistic care.

1. Selective Serotonin Reuptake Inhibitors (SSRIs) for Binge Eating Disorder

Mechanism of Action

SSRIs, commonly used as antidepressants, have demonstrated effectiveness in treating binge eating disorder. The mechanism of action involves increasing serotonin levels in the brain, which can modulate mood and appetite regulation. By targeting the emotional aspects linked to binge eating, SSRIs contribute to symptom reduction.

Commonly Prescribed SSRIs

- **Fluoxetine (Prozac):** Prozac, a widely prescribed SSRI, has shown efficacy in reducing binge eating episodes and promoting emotional well-being.

- **Sertraline (Zoloft):** Zoloft is another SSRI that has demonstrated benefits in addressing the emotional components associated with binge eating disorder.

2. Serotonin-Norepinephrine Reuptake Inhibitors (SNRIs) and Binge Eating

Expanding the Neurotransmitter Scope

SNRIs, like SSRIs, impact neurotransmitter levels but target both serotonin and norepinephrine. While not specifically FDA-approved for binge eating disorder, some SNRIs may be considered off-label for their potential benefits in addressing mood and emotional factors associated with binge eating.

Potential Medications

- **Venlafaxine (Effexor):** Effexor, an SNRI, is sometimes explored for its impact on emotional regulation, although its use for binge eating disorder is off-label.

3. Topiramate: Targeting Neurological Pathways

Antiepileptic Properties

Topiramate, an antiepileptic medication, has demonstrated efficacy in reducing binge eating episodes. Its neurological impact is thought to influence appetite regulation and impulse control, making it a consideration for individuals with binge eating disorder.

Considerations and Side Effects

- **Weight Loss:** Topiramate is associated with weight loss, which may be beneficial for individuals with binge eating disorder who are also concerned about weight management.
- **Cognitive Effects:** Some individuals may experience cognitive side effects,

requiring careful consideration and monitoring.

4. Naltrexone and Binge Eating Disorder

<u>Opioid Receptor Blockade</u>

Naltrexone, primarily used to manage opioid and alcohol dependence, has shown promise in reducing binge eating episodes. By blocking opioid receptors, naltrexone may influence the reward system associated with food, contributing to a decrease in binge eating behaviors.

Potential Medications

- **Naltrexone-Bupropion (Contrave):** Contrave, a combination of naltrexone and bupropion, is an FDA-approved medication for weight management that may be considered for individuals with binge eating disorder.

5. Lisdexamfetamine: Stimulant Medication for Binge Eating

<u>Amphetamine Derivative</u>

Lisdexamfetamine, an amphetamine derivative, is FDA-approved for the treatment of binge eating disorder. It works by affecting neurotransmitters in the brain, influencing impulse control and reducing the frequency of binge eating episodes.

<u>Considerations and Monitoring</u>

- *Cardiovascular Effects:* Due to its stimulant nature, lisdexamfetamine requires careful monitoring for potential cardiovascular effects.
- *Abuse Potential:* Individuals with a history of substance abuse may need

cautious consideration when prescribing stimulant medications.

6. Collaborative Care and Monitoring

Holistic Approach

The use of medications for binge eating disorder is often integrated into a comprehensive treatment plan that includes psychotherapy, lifestyle modifications, and nutritional guidance. Collaborative care ensures that individuals receive personalized and well-rounded support.

Monitoring and Adjustments

Regular monitoring by healthcare professionals is crucial to assess the effectiveness and side effects of medications. Adjustments to the medication plan may be made based on an individual's response and evolving needs during the course of treatment.

Conclusion

Medications play a significant role in the multifaceted approach to managing binge eating disorder. While they are not standalone solutions, medications, when carefully prescribed and monitored, can contribute to symptom reduction and provide valuable support in the journey toward recovery. The decision to use medications should be made collaboratively between individuals and healthcare professionals, considering the unique aspects of each person's experience with binge eating disorder.

The Role of Healthcare Professionals in Binge Eating Disorder

In the complex landscape of binge eating disorder (BED), the role of healthcare professionals is paramount in orchestrating comprehensive and personalized care. From diagnosis to treatment planning, healthcare professionals bring expertise, guidance, and support to individuals navigating the challenges of BED. This section explores the multifaceted contributions of healthcare professionals, encompassing diagnosis, collaboration in treatment, monitoring, and the holistic care necessary for lasting recovery.

1. Diagnosis and Assessment by Healthcare Professionals

Specialized Evaluation

The journey toward recovery begins with accurate diagnosis. Healthcare professionals, including psychiatrists, psychologists, and primary care physicians, play a crucial role in conducting a specialized evaluation. They assess symptoms, explore the emotional and psychological aspects of binge eating, and consider contributing factors such as co-occurring mental health conditions.

Differential Diagnosis

Healthcare professionals distinguish BED from other eating disorders, ensuring a precise diagnosis. Differential diagnosis involves considering conditions such as bulimia nervosa, anorexia nervosa, and other mental health disorders with overlapping features. Accurate diagnosis forms the foundation for tailored treatment strategies.

2. Collaborative Treatment Planning

Integrated Care Teams

The treatment of BED often involves a collaborative approach. Healthcare professionals collaborate with a diverse team, including therapists, dietitians, and other specialists, to formulate comprehensive treatment plans. This collaborative effort addresses the biological, psychological, and social aspects of BED, ensuring a holistic and individualized approach.

Psychotherapy and Medication Integration

Healthcare professionals coordinate the integration of psychotherapy and, when deemed appropriate, medications. Psychotherapy, including Cognitive-Behavioral Therapy (CBT),

Dialectical Behavior Therapy (DBT), and Interpersonal Psychotherapy (IPT), addresses the psychological aspects of BED. Medications, such as selective serotonin reuptake inhibitors (SSRIs) or stimulants, may be prescribed to complement psychotherapeutic interventions.

3. Regular Monitoring and Adjustment

Health Checkups and Laboratory Assessments

Healthcare professionals oversee regular health checkups and laboratory assessments to monitor physical health. Binge eating can have implications for cardiovascular health, metabolic function, and nutritional status. Monitoring provides a comprehensive view of an individual's well-being and guides adjustments to the treatment plan as needed.

<u>Medication Management</u>

For individuals prescribed medications, healthcare professionals manage the ongoing assessment of medication effectiveness and potential side effects. Adjustments to medication regimens are made based on individual responses, ensuring optimal therapeutic outcomes while minimizing adverse effects.

4. Nutritional Guidance and Dietetics

<u>Registered Dietitian Involvement</u>

Healthcare professionals collaborate with registered dietitians to provide nutritional guidance. Dietitians play a crucial role in addressing the dietary aspects of BED, helping individuals establish balanced eating patterns, manage triggers, and cultivate a healthy relationship with food.

<u>Individualized Meal Planning</u>

Healthcare professionals, alongside dietitians, contribute to individualized meal planning. Tailored nutritional plans consider an individual's preferences, cultural factors, and nutritional needs, fostering a sustainable and nourishing approach to eating.

5. Mental Health Support and Counseling

<u>Therapeutic Interventions</u>

In collaboration with therapists and mental health professionals, healthcare providers offer ongoing mental health support. Therapeutic interventions address the emotional aspects of BED, including stress management, coping skills development, and exploring the root causes of binge eating behaviors.

<u>Crisis Intervention and Urgent Care</u>

Healthcare professionals are equipped to provide crisis intervention and urgent care for individuals facing acute episodes or crises related to BED. Timely support and intervention during challenging moments are integral components of comprehensive care.

6. Educational Guidance and Community Resources

Informative Sessions

Healthcare professionals engage in educational guidance, offering informative sessions to individuals and their families. These sessions cover topics such as the nature of BED, available treatment options, and strategies for building a supportive environment. Education fosters awareness and empowers individuals in their journey toward recovery.

Connecting with Community Resources

Healthcare professionals assist individuals in connecting with community resources, support groups, and online communities. These resources provide additional avenues for ongoing support, fostering a sense of community and reducing feelings of isolation.

Conclusion

The role of healthcare professionals in the treatment of binge eating disorder extends beyond diagnosis to encompass comprehensive care. By collaborating with a diverse team, monitoring physical and mental health, and providing tailored interventions, healthcare professionals contribute significantly to the journey of individuals striving for lasting recovery. The orchestration of care by healthcare professionals reflects a commitment to addressing the multifaceted aspects of BED and fostering the well-being of those affected by this challenging disorder.

Chapter 7

Self-Help Strategies

In the pursuit of overcoming binge eating, empowerment lies not only in professional interventions but also in the strength of self-help strategies.

In this chapter, you are going to discover and learn

1. Building a Support System

   ★ Friends, Family, and Community

   ★ Online Support Groups

2. Nutritional Education and Planning

   ★ Balancing Nutrition for Mental and Physical Well-being

   ★ Meal Planning and Preparation Tips

Building a Support System

Embarking on the path to overcome binge eating is not a solitary journey. In this chapter, we delve into the transformative power of building a support system – a network of pillars comprising friends, family, and community. As we explore the significance of these connections and the dynamic realm of online support groups, discover how these foundations become instrumental in fostering understanding, empathy, and encouragement. Together, we unravel the strength found in shared experiences and mutual support, laying the groundwork for a resilient and empowering journey towards recovery.

Friend

Anchors of Understanding and Encouragement in Overcoming Binge Eating

In the challenging journey to overcome binge eating, the role of friends transcends mere companionship; they become anchors of understanding and encouragement. Friends, when informed and supportive, contribute significantly to an individual's emotional well-being and recovery process. This section explores the multifaceted ways in which friends can provide valuable support, foster empathy, and create a nurturing environment conducive to healing from binge eating disorder.

1. Understanding the Nature of Binge Eating

<u>Education and Awareness</u>

In the realm of supporting a friend dealing with binge eating, knowledge is a powerful ally. Friends who take the initiative to educate themselves about the nature of binge eating disorder demonstrate a level of understanding that forms the foundation for meaningful support. This education involves learning about the emotional, psychological, and physical aspects of binge eating.

<u>Open Communication</u>

Understanding begins with open communication. Friends who create a safe space for their loved ones to share their experiences, thoughts, and struggles foster an environment where individuals feel heard and supported. This open dialogue is essential for dismantling stigmas and fostering a culture of empathy.

2. Providing Emotional Support

<u>Non-Judgmental Listening</u>

One of the most impactful ways friends can support individuals dealing with binge eating is through non-judgmental listening. Being present without criticism or judgment allows individuals to express their feelings and challenges freely. This empathetic listening fosters a sense of validation and reduces feelings of isolation.

<u>Empathy and Validation</u>

Empathy is a key component of emotional support. Friends who can empathize with the emotional struggles associated with binge eating provide a powerful source of validation. Acknowledging the difficulties without minimizing or dismissing feelings helps individuals feel understood and accepted.

3. Assisting in Seeking Professional Help

Encouraging Professional Guidance

Friends play a crucial role in encouraging their loved ones to seek professional help. Whether suggesting therapy, counseling, or consultation with a healthcare professional, friends act as advocates for the importance of expert guidance in the journey toward recovery. Encouragement can be a motivating factor for individuals to take the step towards seeking professional assistance.

Supporting Treatment Plans

Once professional help is initiated, friends can further support their loved ones by actively engaging in the treatment process. This may involve attending therapy sessions together, providing transportation to appointments, or offering encouragement to adhere to treatment plans. A supportive friend presence enhances the effectiveness of therapeutic interventions.

4. Creating a Nurturing Environment

<u>Positive Reinforcement</u>

Friends contribute to a nurturing environment by providing positive reinforcement. Celebrating small victories, acknowledging progress, and expressing confidence in an individual's ability to overcome challenges contribute to a positive atmosphere that bolsters self-esteem and resilience.

<u>Participating in Healthy Activities</u>

Engaging in healthy activities together promotes a balanced and supportive lifestyle. Friends can suggest and participate in activities that foster physical and mental well-being, such as exercise, outdoor adventures, or creative pursuits. These activities provide alternative outlets for stress and contribute to overall wellness.

5. Encouraging Self-Care Practices

<u>Promoting Healthy Self-Care Habits</u>

Friends play a pivotal role in encouraging self-care practices. Whether it's advocating for adequate sleep, balanced nutrition, or engaging in activities that bring joy, friends contribute to a holistic approach to well-being. Prioritizing self-care enhances an individual's ability to cope with stressors without resorting to maladaptive behaviors like binge eating.

<u>Being Mindful of Triggers</u>

Understanding and being mindful of potential triggers is crucial for friends supporting individuals with binge eating disorder. Friends can actively contribute to creating a trigger-aware environment by avoiding situations or conversations that may exacerbate stress or anxiety.

Conclusion

Friends serve as anchors of understanding and encouragement in the journey to overcome binge eating. By fostering open communication, providing emotional support, actively participating in the treatment process, and creating a nurturing environment, friends become instrumental allies. Their unwavering support contributes to the resilience and strength needed for individuals to navigate the complexities of binge eating disorder and work towards lasting recovery.

Friends, Family, and Community

Family

The family unit stands as a foundational pillar of support, playing a crucial role in the journey to overcome binge eating. In this exploration, we delve into the multifaceted ways in which families can become catalysts for understanding, empathy, and resilience. From education about binge eating disorder to fostering open communication, families become integral allies in the pursuit of lasting recovery. This comprehensive guide outlines the avenues through which families can provide unwavering support while navigating the challenges associated with binge eating disorder.

1. Educating the Family about Binge Eating Disorder

Knowledge as Empowerment

The journey begins with knowledge. Families actively involved in educating themselves about binge eating disorder empower themselves to become informed allies. Understanding the emotional, psychological, and physical aspects of the disorder allows family members to provide empathetic and effective support.

Shared Learning Experience

Educational initiatives become a shared learning experience for families. Engaging in discussions about the nature of binge eating, its potential triggers, and the impact on mental health fosters an environment where everyone can contribute to the collective understanding. This shared knowledge becomes the foundation for empathy and solidarity.

2. Fostering Open Communication within the Family

Creating a Safe Space

Open communication is the cornerstone of familial support. Families that create a safe and non-judgmental space for individuals to express their thoughts and feelings facilitate an atmosphere where open dialogue can flourish. This safe space is vital for individuals to share their experiences, challenges, and aspirations without fear of criticism.

Encouraging Expressiveness

Encouraging expressiveness within the family dynamic involves validating and acknowledging emotions. Family members who actively listen, ask open-ended questions, and express empathy contribute to an environment where individuals feel heard and understood. This encouragement fosters a sense of emotional safety.

3. Active Involvement in Treatment Plans

Collaborative Treatment Approach

Families can actively participate in the treatment process by adopting a collaborative approach. This involves attending therapy sessions together, engaging in family therapy if recommended, and supporting the implementation of treatment plans. A united front in the pursuit of recovery enhances the effectiveness of therapeutic interventions.

Supporting Lifestyle Modifications

Beyond psychotherapy, families can support lifestyle modifications that contribute to overall well-being. This may include participating in physical activities together, adopting balanced nutritional practices, and creating an environment that promotes mental health. Shared lifestyle adjustments reinforce a sense of unity and commitment to positive change.

4. Promoting Emotional Support and Understanding

Providing Unconditional Support

Emotional support from family members becomes a powerful source of strength. Families that offer unconditional support, regardless of setbacks or challenges, create a foundation on which individuals can build resilience. This unwavering support is integral in navigating the ups and downs of the recovery journey.

Understanding the Emotional Struggles

Family members who actively seek to understand the emotional struggles associated with binge eating demonstrate empathy. Recognizing the impact of stress, anxiety, and emotional distress on binge eating behaviors allows families to offer support that addresses the root causes of the disorder.

5. Creating a Structured and Nurturing Environment

Establishing Routine and Predictability

A structured environment contributes to stability, which is particularly beneficial for individuals dealing with binge eating disorder. Families can create routines that provide predictability, reducing uncertainty and anxiety. Consistency in daily life helps individuals feel secure and supported.

<u>Nurturing Emotional Wellness</u>

Families play a pivotal role in nurturing emotional wellness. This involves promoting activities that bring joy, fostering a positive atmosphere, and actively participating in each other's emotional well-being. Emotional nurturing contributes to a resilient mindset, aiding individuals in coping with stressors without resorting to maladaptive behaviors.

6. Setting Boundaries and Recognizing Triggers

<u>Establishing Healthy Boundaries</u>

Setting and respecting healthy boundaries is crucial for families supporting individuals with binge eating disorder. Recognizing the importance of personal space, privacy, and autonomy contributes to a respectful and supportive family dynamic.

Identifying and Addressing Triggers

Families can collaborate with individuals to identify potential triggers for binge eating episodes. Whether related to stress, interpersonal dynamics, or environmental factors, recognizing triggers allows families to actively address these issues and create a supportive environment that minimizes potential stressors.

Conclusion

Families emerge as pillars of support and resilience in the battle against binge eating. By fostering open communication, actively participating in treatment plans, providing emotional support, creating a nurturing environment, and recognizing the importance of boundaries, families contribute significantly to the journey of recovery. Their commitment to understanding, empathy, and collaborative support becomes a guiding force in helping individuals navigate the complexities of binge eating disorder and build a foundation for lasting well-being.

Community

In the journey to overcome binge eating, the broader community serves as a vital source of strength, understanding, and shared experiences. This section explores the multifaceted role of community support in fostering resilience and contributing to the collective healing of individuals dealing with binge eating disorder. From local initiatives to online forums, the community becomes a dynamic space where empathy, encouragement, and shared wisdom converge, creating an environment conducive to lasting recovery.

1. Local Support Initiatives and Groups

Community-Centric Support Groups

Local communities often host support groups specifically tailored for individuals dealing with binge eating disorder. These groups provide a safe and non-judgmental space where individuals can share their experiences, challenges, and successes. Community-centric support initiatives facilitate connections with others who understand the nuances of binge eating, fostering a sense of belonging.

Educational Workshops and Events

Communities may organize educational workshops and events to raise awareness about binge eating disorder. These initiatives not only contribute to destigmatizing the disorder but also empower individuals with knowledge about available resources and effective coping strategies. The exchange of information within the community becomes a catalyst for understanding and empathy.

2. Online Support Forums and Communities

Virtual Connections

In the digital age, online support forums and communities play a pivotal role in connecting individuals worldwide. These virtual spaces provide a platform for sharing personal stories, seeking advice, and offering encouragement. Online communities create a global network of support, ensuring that individuals have access to diverse perspectives and coping strategies.

<u>Real-Time Support</u>

The immediacy of online communication enables real-time support. Individuals can reach out for assistance, share their struggles, or offer guidance at any moment. This instantaneous connectivity fosters a sense of community that transcends geographical boundaries, creating a virtual haven for those navigating the challenges of binge eating disorder.

3. Peer Mentoring and Sponsorship Programs

<u>Peer-to-Peer Support Networks</u>

Communities may establish peer mentoring programs where individuals further along in their recovery journey provide support to those at earlier stages. Peer-to-peer connections offer unique insights and understanding, as mentors share personal experiences and strategies that have been effective for them. This reciprocal support strengthens the fabric of the community.

Sponsorship for Accountability

Sponsorship programs involve individuals with more extensive recovery experience guiding and supporting those in the early stages of their journey. The sponsorship dynamic fosters accountability, encouragement, and a sense of responsibility within the community. These structured relationships contribute to a supportive framework for long-term recovery.

4. Community-Driven Events and Activities

Wellness Workshops and Retreats

Communities may organize wellness workshops and retreats that focus on various aspects of health, including mental well-being and nutritional education. These events provide opportunities for individuals to engage in supportive activities, learn new coping skills, and connect with like-minded peers in a positive and nurturing environment.

Recreational and Social Gatherings

In addition to formal events, communities may arrange recreational and social gatherings that emphasize building connections and fostering a sense of camaraderie. These casual interactions contribute to the development of a supportive community where individuals feel understood, accepted, and valued.

5. Advocacy and Awareness Initiatives

Community-Led Advocacy

Communities can play a pivotal role in advocating for increased awareness and understanding of binge eating disorder. Community-led initiatives may involve collaboration with local organizations, educational institutions, and healthcare providers to promote awareness campaigns, destigmatize the disorder, and encourage early intervention.

Reducing Stigma and Fostering Compassion

Community-driven efforts to reduce stigma contribute to creating an environment where individuals feel comfortable seeking help. By fostering compassion and understanding, communities become catalysts for change, actively participating in the collective mission to address the challenges associated with binge eating disorder.

6. Access to Resources and Professional Guidance

Community Resource Centers

Communities may establish resource centers that provide access to information, educational materials, and resources related to binge eating disorder. These centers serve as hubs for individuals seeking support, guidance, and reliable information about treatment options, nutritional counseling, and local support groups.

Collaboration with Healthcare Professionals

Community initiatives often involve collaboration with healthcare professionals to ensure individuals receive comprehensive support. This collaboration may include hosting workshops led by mental health experts, organizing outreach programs, and facilitating connections between community members and healthcare providers.

<u>**Conclusion**</u>

Community support becomes a linchpin in the journey toward recovery from binge eating disorder. Whether through local support groups, online forums, peer mentoring programs, or community-driven events, the collective strength of the community fosters understanding, empathy, and shared wisdom. In the embrace of a supportive community, individuals find the encouragement and resilience needed to navigate the complexities of binge eating disorder and embark on a path toward lasting well-being.

Online Support Groups

In the digital era, online support groups emerge as transformative spaces where individuals dealing with binge eating disorder find solace, understanding, and a sense of community. This section explores the profound impact of online support groups in fostering connection, providing real-time support, and creating a global network of shared experiences. From the dynamics of virtual communication to the diverse perspectives within these groups, discover how these online havens become pillars of strength in the journey toward recovery.

1. Global Reach and Diverse Perspectives

Connecting Across Boundaries

One of the primary strengths of online support groups lies in their ability to connect individuals from diverse geographical locations. This global reach ensures that individuals have access to a wide spectrum of perspectives, experiences, and coping strategies. The diversity within these groups enriches the collective knowledge and understanding of binge eating disorder.

Cultural Sensitivity and Inclusivity

Online support groups foster a sense of inclusivity by accommodating individuals from various cultural backgrounds. This cultural sensitivity creates an environment where diverse experiences are acknowledged and respected. Participants can share how cultural factors may influence their relationship with food and contribute unique insights to the group dynamic.

2. Real-Time Support and Immediate Connectivity

24/7 Accessibility

Unlike traditional support structures, online groups offer continuous accessibility.

Participants can seek support, share experiences, or offer encouragement at any time, creating a dynamic and responsive support system. This real-time connectivity addresses the immediate needs of individuals dealing with the challenges of binge eating disorder.

Instantaneous Peer Support

The immediacy of virtual communication allows for instantaneous peer support. Participants can share their struggles, celebrate victories, or seek advice in real time. This instantaneous connectivity fosters a sense of camaraderie and understanding, creating a virtual space where individuals feel heard and supported.

3. Anonymity and Confidentiality

Creating a Safe Space

Online support groups often provide a level of anonymity that may be comforting for individuals hesitant to share their experiences in a face-to-face setting. This anonymity creates a safe space where participants can express themselves without fear of judgment or stigma. Confidentiality within the group ensures a protective environment for personal narratives.

Overcoming Stigmas

The ability to participate without revealing one's identity can be empowering for those contending with stigmas associated with binge eating disorder. Anonymity allows individuals to focus on shared experiences, coping strategies, and mutual support, fostering a collective sense of empowerment in overcoming societal biases.

4. **Structured Group Dynamics**

Facilitated Discussions and Themes

Online support groups often have structured discussions facilitated by moderators or group leaders. These discussions may revolve around specific themes, coping strategies, or challenges associated with binge eating disorder. This structured approach ensures that group interactions are purposeful and contribute to the overall well-being of participants.

Individualized Interaction

Participants in online support groups have the flexibility to engage in both group discussions and individualized interactions. This dynamic allows individuals to receive personalized support, share their unique experiences, and form connections with others who may be navigating similar aspects of binge eating disorder.

5. Resource Sharing and Educational Opportunities

Access to Information

Online support groups serve as valuable hubs for sharing resources and educational materials. Participants can access information about the latest research, treatment options, and self-help strategies related to binge eating disorder. This resource-sharing dynamic empowers individuals with knowledge to make informed decisions about their recovery journey.

Guest Speakers and Experts

Some online groups may organize sessions with guest speakers or experts in the field of binge eating disorder. These sessions provide participants with the opportunity to learn from professionals, ask questions, and gain insights into various aspects of the disorder. Educational opportunities within the online space contribute to a holistic approach to recovery.

6. Mutual Accountability and Encouragement

Setting Goals and Milestones

Online support groups often incorporate elements of mutual accountability. Participants can set personal goals and milestones, sharing them with the group for encouragement and support. The collective encouragement and celebration of achievements create a motivating atmosphere within the virtual community.

Daily Check-Ins and Progress Updates

Regular check-ins and progress updates become integral components of online support groups. Participants can share their daily experiences, challenges, and successes, receiving encouragement and insights from others. This ongoing exchange fosters a sense of community and mutual accountability that contributes to individual resilience.

Conclusion

Online support groups, with their global reach, real-time connectivity, and emphasis on anonymity, form an integral part of the support landscape for individuals dealing with binge eating disorder. By providing a virtual haven of understanding, encouragement, and shared wisdom, these groups empower individuals to navigate the complexities of their journey toward recovery. In the dynamic realm of online support, participants find strength in collective resilience and the unwavering support of a global community.

Nutritional Education and Planning

In the intricate tapestry of overcoming binge eating, nutritional education and planning emerge as keystones for fostering a harmonious relationship between the mind and body. This section explores the transformative power of understanding the role of nutrition in mental well-being. From balanced dietary practices to personalized meal planning, embark on a journey that not only nourishes the body but also contributes to a holistic approach to mental health and recovery.

Balancing Nutrition for Mental and Physical Well-being

The Intersection of Nourishment and Mental Health

In the intricate dance between nutritional choices and overall well-being, finding a harmonious balance is key to fostering mental and physical health. This section delves into the profound impact of balanced nutrition on mental well-being, exploring how the foods we consume can influence mood, cognitive function, and emotional resilience. From essential nutrients that support brain health to the concept of mindful eating, discover the nuanced interplay between nutrition and mental flourishing.

1. Essential Nutrients for Brain Health

Omega-3 Fatty Acids

Omega-3 fatty acids, found in fatty fish, flaxseeds, and walnuts, play a crucial role in supporting brain health. These essential fats contribute to the structural integrity of brain cells and are associated with cognitive function and emotional well-being. Including omega-3-rich foods in the diet can be a nutritional cornerstone for mental wellness.

Antioxidants

Antioxidant-rich foods, such as berries, dark leafy greens, and nuts, protect the brain from oxidative stress. These compounds combat inflammation and may contribute to the prevention of mental decline. Integrating a variety of colorful, antioxidant-packed foods into the diet supports both mental and physical resilience.

2. Blood Sugar Regulation and Mood Stability

Complex Carbohydrates

Balancing blood sugar levels is pivotal for mood stability. Complex carbohydrates, like whole grains, legumes, and vegetables, provide a steady release of glucose, preventing energy crashes and mood swings. Prioritizing complex carbs in meals contributes to sustained mental alertness and emotional balance.

Protein-Rich Foods

Including adequate protein in the diet supports stable blood sugar levels and promotes feelings of fullness. Protein sources such as lean meats, beans, and tofu contribute to the synthesis of neurotransmitters like dopamine and serotonin, influencing mood regulation.

3. The Gut-Brain Connection

Probiotics and Fermented Foods

The gut-brain connection highlights the profound impact of gut health on mental well-being. Probiotics, found in fermented foods like yogurt, kefir, and sauerkraut, support a healthy gut microbiome. A balanced gut microbiome is associated with improved mood and reduced symptoms of anxiety and depression.

Fiber-Rich Foods

Fiber, abundant in fruits, vegetables, and whole grains, nourishes the gut microbiota. A diverse and thriving microbiome is linked to enhanced mental resilience. Prioritizing fiber-rich foods supports both digestive health and the intricate interplay between gut and brain function.

4. Mindful Eating Practices

<u>Cultivating Awareness</u>

Mindful eating involves cultivating awareness of the present moment while consuming food. This practice encourages individuals to savor flavors, textures, and aromas, fostering a deeper connection with the act of eating. By being present during meals, individuals can better tune into hunger and fullness cues, promoting a balanced approach to nutrition.

<u>Emotional Eating Awareness</u>

Mindful eating also addresses emotional eating by promoting awareness of the emotions tied to food consumption. Recognizing emotional triggers allows individuals to make conscious choices about when and what to eat, breaking the cycle of using food as a coping mechanism for stress or emotional distress.

5. Hydration and Cognitive Function

Water as a Cognitive Enhancer

Proper hydration is fundamental for optimal cognitive function. Dehydration can impair attention, memory, and mood. Ensuring an adequate intake of water throughout the day supports mental alertness and overall cognitive performance.

Limiting Dehydrating Substances

Conversely, reducing the consumption of dehydrating substances such as caffeine and alcohol supports hydration. Excessive intake of these substances can contribute to dehydration, impacting mental clarity and contributing to feelings of fatigue.

6. Individualized Meal Planning for Mental Well-being

Personalized Nutrition Plans

Recognizing the individuality of nutritional needs, personalized meal planning takes into account factors such as age, gender, activity level, and specific health considerations. Tailoring nutrition plans to individual requirements ensures that dietary choices support both mental and physical well-being.

Collaboration with Nutrition Professionals

Working with nutrition professionals, such as registered dietitians, provides individuals with expert guidance in crafting personalized meal plans. These professionals can assess nutritional needs, address specific concerns, and offer practical strategies for incorporating balanced and nourishing meals into daily life.

Conclusion

The intricate interplay between nutrition and mental well-being underscores the importance of balanced dietary practices. From essential nutrients that support brain health to mindful eating practices and individualized meal planning, the choices we make in nourishing our bodies have a profound impact on our mental and physical resilience. As we navigate the delicate dance of balancing nutrition for well-being, we empower ourselves to cultivate a holistic approach to mental health and embark on a journey of sustained vitality.

Meal Planning and Preparation Tips

Embarking on a journey of balanced nutrition involves thoughtful meal planning and preparation. This section delves into practical strategies and tips for creating nourishing meals that support both mental and physical well-being. From organizing weekly menus to incorporating diverse food groups, discover the key elements of effective meal planning and preparation that contribute to a sustainable and healthful lifestyle.

1. Establishing a Weekly Meal Routine

Designing a Balanced Menu

Begin the meal planning process by designing a balanced menu for the week. Ensure a variety of food groups are included, incorporating fruits, vegetables, lean proteins, whole grains, and healthy fats. This diversity ensures a broad range of nutrients that contribute to overall well-being.

Consideration of Dietary Preferences and Restrictions

Tailor the menu to individual dietary preferences and restrictions. Whether following specific dietary guidelines, accommodating food allergies, or exploring cultural preferences, a personalized approach to meal planning enhances satisfaction and adherence to nutritional goals.

2. Efficient Grocery Shopping Strategies

Creating a Detailed Shopping List

Before heading to the grocery store, create a detailed shopping list based on the planned meals. This list helps streamline the shopping process, reduces impulse purchases, and ensures all necessary ingredients are available for meal preparation.

Choosing Fresh and Whole Foods

Prioritize fresh, whole foods when selecting items for your meals. Opt for a colorful array of fruits and vegetables, lean proteins, whole grains, and minimally processed items. These choices contribute to a nutrient-dense and healthful diet.

3. Prepping Ingredients for Convenience

Batch Prepping Staples

Simplify meal preparation by batch prepping staple ingredients. Cook and portion items like grains, proteins, and vegetables in advance, storing them for quick and convenient use throughout the week. Batch prepping enhances efficiency and encourages consistency in meal choices.

Washing and Chopping Produce

Allocate time to wash and chop fruits and vegetables when returning from the grocery store. Prepped produce is easily accessible for snacking or incorporation into meals, promoting a higher intake of nutrient-rich foods.

4. Mindful Portion Control

Using Portion-Controlled Containers

Invest in portion-controlled containers to assist in mindful eating practices. Preparing meals in these containers supports portion control, helping to avoid overeating and ensuring a well-balanced intake of nutrients.

Balancing Macronutrients

When planning meals, consider the balance of macronutrients—proteins, carbohydrates, and fats. Aim for a distribution that aligns with individual dietary needs and supports sustained energy levels throughout the day.

5. Diversifying Culinary Techniques

<u>Exploring Various Cooking Methods</u>

Diversify your culinary techniques by exploring various cooking methods. Incorporate grilled, roasted, steamed, and sautéed options to add variety to meals. Experimenting with different methods enhances the sensory experience of eating and keeps meals interesting.

<u>Incorporating Herbs and Spices</u>

Enhance the flavor profile of meals by incorporating a variety of herbs and spices. Experimenting with different seasonings adds depth and complexity to dishes without relying on excessive salt or sugar, contributing to a healthful and enjoyable dining experience.

6. Sustainable and Flexible Meal Plans

<u>Adapting to Changing Schedules</u>

Create meal plans that are flexible and adaptable to changing schedules. Account for busy days by incorporating quick and easy recipes, and plan for leftovers that can be repurposed into subsequent meals. This adaptability fosters consistency in maintaining a balanced diet.

<u>Reducing Food Waste</u>

Minimize food waste by strategically planning meals that use overlapping ingredients. Incorporate perishable items earlier in the week and frozen or longer-lasting items later. Staying mindful of expiration dates and repurposing leftovers contributes to sustainability.

7. Prioritizing Hydration

Incorporating Hydrating Foods

Include hydrating foods, such as water-rich fruits and vegetables, as part of meal planning. These foods contribute to overall hydration levels, supporting cognitive function and physical well-being. Additionally, prioritize regular water intake throughout the day.

Limiting Sugary Beverages

When considering beverage options, limit the consumption of sugary drinks. Opt for water, herbal teas, or infused water to reduce added sugars in the diet. Adequate hydration is essential for optimal mental and physical performance.

<u>Conclusion</u>

Crafting nourishing routines through effective meal planning and preparation is a foundational step towards achieving both mental and physical well-being. By establishing a weekly meal routine, adopting efficient grocery shopping strategies, prepping ingredients for convenience, practicing mindful portion control, diversifying culinary techniques, creating sustainable meal plans, and prioritizing hydration, individuals can cultivate a healthful and enjoyable approach to nutrition. Through these practices, mealtime becomes a nourishing ritual that contributes to sustained vitality and supports the journey to holistic well-being.

Chapter 8

Overcoming Triggers

In Chapter 8, we embark on a transformative exploration of overcoming triggers in the pursuit of resilience. This section delves into the intricacies of identifying and managing triggers associated with binge eating disorder. From unveiling the roots of these triggers to developing effective coping strategies, join the journey of building resilience that transcends challenges and paves the way for lasting well-being. It's a narrative of empowerment, self-discovery, and the unwavering strength found in navigating the complex terrain of trigger management.

This chapter, will delve into:

1. Identifying and Managing Triggers
   ★ Developing Coping Strategies
   ★ Building Resilience

Identifying and Managing Triggers

Chapter 8 delves into the profound task of identifying and managing triggers, the intricate threads that weave through the tapestry of binge eating disorder. In this exploration, we navigate the complexities of recognizing the catalysts that lead to maladaptive behaviors. Through heightened awareness and strategic management, individuals embark on a journey of reclaiming control and fostering resilience. Join us in unraveling the threads of influence, understanding triggers, and charting a course towards lasting recovery.

Developing Coping Strategies

In the intricate landscape of overcoming binge eating disorder, developing effective coping strategies stands as a cornerstone for resilience and lasting recovery. This section explores a spectrum of strategies that empower individuals to navigate the challenges associated with triggers and foster a healthy relationship with food. From mindfulness techniques to building a personalized toolbox of coping mechanisms, discover a comprehensive guide to developing coping strategies that transcend adversity.

1. Mindfulness and Grounding Techniques

Mindful Eating Practices

Cultivating mindfulness in eating involves being fully present during meals, savoring each bite, and paying attention to hunger and fullness cues. Mindful eating promotes a conscious and intentional approach to food, reducing the likelihood of impulsive or emotional eating.

Grounding Exercises

Grounding techniques, such as deep breathing, sensory awareness, or visualization, can be powerful tools to bring awareness to the present moment. These exercises assist in redirecting attention away from triggers, helping individuals regain control over their thoughts and emotions.

2. Emotional Regulation and Expression

Emotion-Focused Strategies

Developing coping strategies that address emotional triggers is crucial. Engaging in activities that foster emotional regulation, such as journaling, art therapy, or talking to a supportive friend, provides healthy outlets for processing and expressing emotions without resorting to binge eating.

Identification of Emotional Triggers

Understanding the emotional triggers that contribute to binge eating is a key step in developing effective coping mechanisms. Through self-reflection and heightened awareness, individuals can identify specific emotions or situations that prompt maladaptive responses and work towards proactive solutions.

3. Cognitive Restructuring and Behavioral Interventions

Cognitive-Behavioral Techniques

Cognitive restructuring involves challenging and reframing negative thought patterns associated with binge eating. Techniques from cognitive-behavioral therapy (CBT) can be valuable in changing dysfunctional beliefs and fostering a healthier mindset towards food and body image.

Behavioral Interventions

Implementing behavioral interventions involves consciously modifying behaviors associated with binge eating. This may include creating structured meal plans, incorporating positive reinforcements, and gradually exposing oneself to triggering situations with the support of a therapist.

4. Building a Support Network

Seeking Professional Guidance

Developing coping strategies often involves seeking support from mental health professionals. Therapists, counselors, or support groups provide guidance in exploring and implementing personalized coping mechanisms, fostering a sense of accountability and encouragement.

Connecting with Peers

Building a supportive network of peers who understand the challenges of binge eating disorder is invaluable. Peer support groups or online communities create spaces for shared experiences, mutual encouragement, and the exchange of coping strategies that have proven effective.

5. Stress Reduction Techniques

Incorporating Relaxation Practices

Stress reduction plays a pivotal role in developing coping strategies. Practices such as yoga, meditation, or progressive muscle relaxation can alleviate stress and contribute to emotional well-being, reducing the likelihood of turning to binge eating as a coping mechanism.

Time Management and Prioritization

Effective time management and prioritization of responsibilities contribute to stress reduction. By organizing daily tasks and setting realistic goals, individuals can create a more balanced and manageable lifestyle, minimizing stressors that may trigger binge eating.

6. Self-Care Practices

Nurturing the Mind and Body

Self-care practices are essential in maintaining mental and physical well-being. Engaging in activities that bring joy, relaxation, and fulfillment, whether it's reading, taking a nature walk, or enjoying a hobby, helps build resilience and provides healthier alternatives to cope with stress.

Establishing Boundaries

Developing coping strategies involves recognizing personal limits and establishing boundaries. Learning to say no, setting realistic expectations, and prioritizing self-care contribute to a balanced lifestyle that supports mental and emotional resilience.

Conclusion

Developing coping strategies is a dynamic and personalized journey that empowers individuals to face triggers with resilience and adaptive responses. By incorporating mindfulness techniques, addressing emotional triggers, restructuring cognitive patterns, building a support network, reducing stress, and prioritizing self-care, individuals embark on a path of self-discovery and healing. This comprehensive approach equips individuals with a diverse toolkit to navigate the complexities of binge eating disorder, fostering lasting recovery and a renewed sense of well-being.

Building Resilience

In the pursuit of lasting recovery from binge eating disorder, building resilience emerges as a transformative journey of self-discovery and empowerment. This section explores the multifaceted aspects of resilience, providing a comprehensive guide to fortifying the mental, emotional, and physical foundations necessary for sustained well-being. From cultivating a resilient mindset to embracing life's uncertainties, discover the key elements that contribute to building resilience in the face of challenges.

1. Cultivating a Resilient Mindset

Adopting a Growth Mindset

Cultivating resilience begins with adopting a growth mindset—a belief that challenges are opportunities for learning and growth. Embracing setbacks as part of the journey allows individuals to approach difficulties with a sense of curiosity and a willingness to adapt.

Positive Self-Talk and Affirmations

Building resilience involves fostering positive self-talk and incorporating affirmations. Encouraging and supportive internal dialogue can counteract negative thoughts, promoting a mindset of self-compassion and reinforcing the belief in one's ability to overcome challenges.

2. Embracing Adaptive Coping Mechanisms

Flexibility and Adaptability

Resilience is closely tied to adaptability and flexibility. Embracing change and adjusting to new circumstances without losing a sense of self allows individuals to navigate the uncertainties of life without resorting to maladaptive coping mechanisms.

Learning from Setbacks

Resilience thrives on the ability to learn from setbacks. Viewing challenges as opportunities for growth and self-discovery fosters a mindset that transforms adversity into valuable experiences, contributing to an individual's overall resilience.

3. Building Emotional Resilience

Emotional Regulation Techniques

Emotional resilience involves developing effective emotional regulation techniques. Practices such as mindfulness, deep breathing, and expressive therapies contribute to a healthy relationship with emotions, preventing the escalation of negative feelings that may lead to binge eating.

Acceptance of Emotions

Resilience includes accepting a wide range of emotions without judgment. Recognizing that all emotions are valid and transient allows individuals to respond to emotional triggers with a balanced and adaptive mindset, reducing the likelihood of turning to maladaptive coping mechanisms.

4. Nurturing Social Connections

Building Supportive Relationships

Social connections are integral to resilience. Building and maintaining supportive relationships provide a network of understanding and encouragement. Friends, family, or support groups contribute to a sense of belonging and offer valuable perspectives in times of difficulty.

Communication and Vulnerability

Resilience is enhanced through open communication and vulnerability. Expressing one's thoughts and feelings to trusted individuals fosters a sense of connection and allows for mutual support. Sharing experiences and seeking assistance when needed contribute to a resilient support network.

5. Physical Resilience and Self-Care

Prioritizing Physical Well-being

Physical resilience is interconnected with self-care practices. Prioritizing sleep, engaging in regular physical activity, and maintaining a balanced diet contribute to overall well-being. A healthy body provides a foundation for mental and emotional resilience.

Restorative Activities

Incorporating restorative activities into daily life enhances physical resilience. Activities such as relaxation exercises, meditation, or hobbies that bring joy and relaxation contribute to stress reduction and support the body's ability to recover from challenges.

6. Setting and Achieving Realistic Goals

Setting Incremental Goals

Building resilience involves setting realistic and achievable goals. Breaking larger objectives into smaller, manageable steps allows individuals to celebrate incremental successes, reinforcing a sense of accomplishment and motivation.

Adapting Goals to Circumstances

Resilience embraces adaptability in goal-setting. Recognizing that circumstances may change and adjusting goals accordingly prevents the undue pressure associated with rigid expectations. A flexible approach to goals promotes resilience in the face of unforeseen challenges.

7. Mindfulness and Present-Moment Awareness

Practicing Mindfulness Meditation

Mindfulness meditation fosters present-moment awareness, a cornerstone of resilience. Regular practice allows individuals to cultivate a non-judgmental awareness of thoughts and emotions, enabling a centered response to stressors and challenges.

Grounding Techniques in Daily Life

Incorporating grounding techniques into daily life enhances mindfulness. Whether through mindful breathing, sensory awareness, or daily rituals, these practices anchor individuals in the present moment, contributing to a resilient mindset.

Conclusion

Building resilience is a holistic and dynamic process that encompasses mental, emotional, and physical well-being. By cultivating a resilient mindset, embracing adaptive coping mechanisms, nurturing social connections, prioritizing physical resilience through self-care, setting realistic goals, and practicing mindfulness, individuals equip themselves with the tools necessary to navigate the complexities of recovery from binge eating disorder. In the embrace of resilience, individuals discover their inherent strength to overcome challenges and foster a renewed sense of purpose and well-being.

Chapter 9

Maintaining a Healthy Lifestyle

In Chapter 9, our exploration shifts to the vital realm of maintaining a healthy lifestyle, focusing on the symbiotic relationship between physical and mental well-being. This section unveils the transformative power of integrating exercise into daily life, delving into the connection between physical activity and mental health. From discovering enjoyable and sustainable exercise routines to embracing holistic practices like yoga and meditation, join the journey of nurturing both body and mind for a balanced and flourishing life.

This chapter, will make you understand:

1. Integrating Exercise

> ★ The Connection Between Physical Activity and Mental Health
>
> ★ Finding Enjoyable and Sustainable Exercise Routines

2. Mind-Body Connection

> ★ Holistic Approaches to Well-being
>
> ★ Incorporating Practices like Yoga and Meditation

Integrating Exercise

Chapter 9 sets the stage for a dynamic exploration into the realm of holistic well-being by diving into the transformative power of integrating exercise. This section unravels the intricate connection between physical activity and mental health, inviting readers to discover the joy and sustainability of personalized exercise routines. Join us in embracing the notion that movement is not only a pathway to physical vitality but a cornerstone of mental and emotional flourishing.

The Connection Between Physical Activity and Mental Health

The profound interconnection between physical activity and mental health forms a cornerstone of holistic well-being. This section explores the intricate ways in which engaging in regular exercise positively influences mental and emotional states, contributing to a resilient and flourishing mind.

1. Neurochemical Impact of Exercise

<u>Endorphin Release</u>

Physical activity triggers the release of endorphins, often referred to as the "feel-good" neurotransmitters. These endorphins act as natural mood elevators, reducing feelings of stress and anxiety while promoting a sense of well-being. The neurochemical response to exercise contributes to an immediate uplift in mood.

Serotonin Regulation

Regular exercise also plays a role in the regulation of serotonin levels in the brain. Serotonin, a neurotransmitter associated with mood stability, is often targeted in the treatment of conditions like depression. Exercise enhances serotonin production, contributing to a more positive emotional state.

2. Stress Reduction and Cortisol Management

<u>Stress-Reducing Effects</u>

Engaging in physical activity acts as a powerful stress reliever. Exercise helps to lower the body's stress hormones, such as cortisol, and promotes the release of tension. Regular physical activity provides an outlet for built-up stress, fostering a calmer and more relaxed mental state.

<u>Cortisol Modulation</u>

The relationship between exercise and cortisol extends beyond stress reduction. Consistent physical activity helps regulate cortisol levels, preventing excessive fluctuations associated with chronic stress. Maintaining a balanced cortisol profile contributes to improved mental resilience and emotional well-being.

3. Enhanced Cognitive Function and Neuroplasticity

<u>Improved Cognitive Performance</u>

Physical activity has been linked to improved cognitive function and memory. Exercise increases blood flow to the brain, delivering oxygen and nutrients that support optimal cognitive performance. Regular engagement in physical activity is associated with sharper focus, enhanced learning, and better decision-making.

<u>Neuroplasticity and Brain Health</u>

Exercise promotes neuroplasticity, the brain's ability to adapt and reorganize itself. This adaptability is crucial for mental health, as it supports the formation of new neural connections and the preservation of cognitive function. Incorporating regular exercise into one's routine contributes to long-term brain health.

4. Mood Regulation and Anxiety Management

Balancing Mood Swings

Physical activity plays a role in regulating mood swings and promoting emotional stability. The consistent release of endorphins during exercise helps mitigate mood fluctuations, providing individuals with a more even-keeled emotional state.

Effective Anxiety Management

Exercise has proven to be an effective strategy for managing symptoms of anxiety. The calming effect of physical activity, coupled with the physiological changes it induces, contributes to a reduction in anxiety levels. Incorporating exercise into daily life serves as a proactive approach to anxiety management.

5. Social and Community Aspects of Exercise

Social Connection and Support

Many forms of exercise offer opportunities for social interaction and connection. Whether participating in group classes, sports, or outdoor activities, the social component of exercise contributes to a sense of community and support. Social engagement is a crucial factor in promoting positive mental health.

Reducing Feelings of Isolation

Regular participation in group or community-based exercise fosters a sense of belonging, reducing feelings of isolation. The shared experience of physical activity creates bonds and provides a supportive environment, enhancing mental well-being through social connectedness.

Conclusion

The intricate connection between physical activity and mental health underscores the transformative potential of exercise in nurturing a resilient and flourishing mind. From the neurochemical impact of endorphins and serotonin regulation to stress reduction, cognitive enhancement, mood regulation, and the social aspects of exercise, engaging in regular physical activity emerges as a holistic approach to promoting mental well-being. As we delve into the dynamic relationship between movement and mental health, we discover that each step, lift, or stretch is a profound investment in the vitality of both body and mind.

Finding Enjoyable and Sustainable Exercise Routines

Embarking on a journey of physical well-being involves discovering exercise routines that are both enjoyable and sustainable. This section guides individuals in navigating the diverse landscape of fitness, ensuring that the chosen activities align with personal preferences and can be seamlessly integrated into one's lifestyle.

1. Exploring Diverse Exercise Modalities

Variety as the Spice of Fitness

Discovering enjoyable and sustainable exercise routines begins with exploring a variety of modalities. From cardiovascular activities like running, cycling, or dancing to strength training, yoga, or team sports, diversity in exercise prevents monotony and keeps individuals engaged.

Incorporating Elements of Play

Turning exercise into play transforms the experience. Engaging in activities that feel more like play than a workout, such as recreational sports, hiking, or dance classes, adds an element of enjoyment that contributes to long-term adherence to a fitness routine.

2. Setting Realistic and Personalized Goals

SMART Goal Setting

Establishing realistic and personalized fitness goals is key to sustainability. Using the SMART criteria—Specific, Measurable, Achievable,

Relevant, and Time-bound—ensures that goals are clear, attainable, and tailored to individual capabilities and aspirations.

Celebrating Milestones and Progress

Celebrate achievements along the way, no matter how small. Recognizing and celebrating milestones and progress fosters a positive relationship with exercise, reinforcing the sense of accomplishment and motivating continued commitment.

3. Incorporating Enjoyable Group Activities

Group Fitness Classes

Participating in group fitness classes offers a social and enjoyable dimension to exercise. Whether it's a dance class, spin class, or group training session, the camaraderie and shared experience enhance motivation and enjoyment.

Team Sports and Recreational Leagues

Engaging in team sports or recreational leagues adds a social component to physical activity. The sense of teamwork and friendly competition makes exercise enjoyable and contributes to the formation of lasting fitness habits.

4. Flexible and Adaptive Fitness Plans

Adapting to Lifestyle Changes

Sustainable exercise routines are adaptable to life's fluctuations. Creating flexible plans that can be adjusted based on changes in schedule, priorities, or preferences ensures that exercise remains an integral part of one's routine.

Balancing Intensity and Recovery

Sustainability involves finding the right balance between workout intensity and adequate recovery. Incorporating rest days, varying workout intensity, and listening to the body's signals contribute to a balanced and sustainable exercise routine.

5. Incorporating Everyday Movement

Active Commuting

Finding enjoyable ways to incorporate movement into daily activities promotes sustainability. Whether it's walking or cycling to work, taking the stairs, or opting for active transportation, integrating movement into daily routines contributes to overall physical activity.

Functional Fitness Practices

Functional fitness, which focuses on movements that mimic everyday activities, enhances sustainability. Incorporating exercises that improve flexibility, balance, and strength relevant to daily life ensures that exercise serves a practical purpose.

6. Embracing Technology and Gamification

Fitness Apps and Wearables

Embracing technology can make exercise more enjoyable. Fitness apps and wearables provide tracking, goal-setting, and interactive features that add an element of gamification, turning the pursuit of fitness into an engaging experience.

Gamified Workouts and Challenges

Participating in gamified workouts and challenges introduces an element of fun and competition. Whether it's virtual races, fitness challenges with friends, or fitness games, gamification enhances the enjoyment of exercise.

7. Mind-Body Practices for Enjoyable Exercise

Yoga and Mindful Movement

Mind-body practices like yoga offer a holistic approach to exercise. Incorporating mindful movement, stretching, and relaxation techniques not only contributes to physical well-being but also enhances the overall enjoyment of the exercise experience.

Dance and Expressive Movement

Dance and expressive movement allow for self-expression while providing a cardiovascular workout. Whether through dance classes, dance-based fitness programs, or spontaneous dance sessions, this form of exercise adds joy and creativity to the routine.

Conclusion

Discovering enjoyable and sustainable exercise routines is a personalized and evolving journey. By exploring diverse modalities, setting realistic goals, incorporating group activities, adapting to lifestyle changes, embracing technology, and integrating mind-body practices, individuals can cultivate a positive and enduring relationship with exercise. The key lies in finding activities that resonate with personal preferences and bring a sense of enjoyment, transforming exercise from a routine obligation to a source of lasting well-being.

Mind-Body Connection

Chapter 9 unfolds a part dedicated to the profound intertwining of the mind and body in the realm of holistic well-being. This section, focusing on the mind-body connection, illuminates the transformative power of aligning mental and physical practices. From embracing mindful movement to exploring practices like yoga and meditation, join us in the exploration of a harmonious journey toward a balanced and flourishing existence.

Holistic Approaches to Well-being

Nurturing Mind, Body, and Soul

Holistic well-being transcends the physical and encompasses the intricate interplay of mind, body, and soul. In this exploration, Chapter 9 delves into holistic approaches that foster a comprehensive sense of well-being, incorporating practices that nourish every facet of one's existence.

1. Mindful Movement Practices

Yoga as a Holistic Discipline

Yoga, originating from ancient traditions, stands as a holistic practice that unites breath, movement, and mindfulness. Its multifaceted benefits include increased flexibility, improved strength, enhanced mental clarity, and a deepened mind-body connection. Whether through Hatha, Vinyasa, or Kundalini yoga, the practice harmonizes physical postures with intentional breathwork and meditation.

Tai Chi for Flowing Energy

Tai Chi, an ancient Chinese martial art, embodies a holistic approach to well-being. Characterized by slow, deliberate movements and focused breath control, Tai Chi promotes balance, flexibility, and the flow of vital energy, known as Qi. Its meditative nature cultivates a sense of calmness and mental clarity.

2. Meditative Practices for Inner Harmony

Mindfulness Meditation for Present Awareness

Mindfulness meditation serves as a powerful tool for cultivating present-moment awareness. By anchoring attention to the breath, sensations, or a focal point, individuals can foster a calm and focused mind. The practice extends beyond formal sessions, encouraging the integration of mindfulness into daily activities for sustained well-being.

Guided Imagery and Visualization

Guided imagery and visualization tap into the mind's creative power. By engaging in mental journeys that evoke positive images and sensations, individuals can promote relaxation, reduce stress, and enhance overall well-being. This holistic approach combines the benefits of imagination and mental focus.

3. Energy Healing Modalities

Reiki for Energetic Balance

Reiki, a Japanese energy healing technique, operates on the premise of balancing the body's energy flow. Practitioners channel universal life energy through their hands, promoting relaxation and facilitating the body's natural healing processes. This holistic modality addresses both physical and energetic dimensions for overall well-being.

Acupuncture and Traditional Chinese Medicine

Acupuncture, rooted in Traditional Chinese Medicine, involves the insertion of thin needles into specific points on the body to stimulate energy flow. This holistic approach promotes balance in the body's vital forces (Qi) and addresses various physical and emotional imbalances, contributing to overall well-being.

4. Nutritional Practices for Mind and Body

Mindful Eating for Conscious Nourishment

Holistic well-being extends to nutritional practices, with mindful eating serving as a foundational approach. By paying attention to hunger cues, savoring flavors, and cultivating a conscious relationship with food, individuals nourish not only the body but also the mind, fostering a balanced and sustainable approach to nutrition.

<u>Nutritional Psychiatry and Mood Influence</u>

Nutritional psychiatry explores the intricate link between diet and mental health. Incorporating nutrient-dense foods rich in omega-3 fatty acids, vitamins, and minerals can positively impact mood and cognitive function. This holistic perspective recognizes the role of nutrition in promoting mental and emotional well-being.

5. Nature Connection and Grounding Practices

<u>Ecopsychology and Nature Immersion</u>

Holistic well-being embraces the healing power of nature. Ecopsychology explores the connection between individuals and the natural environment, recognizing the therapeutic benefits of immersing oneself in nature. Whether through forest bathing, nature walks, or outdoor meditation, this holistic approach nurtures mental and emotional resilience.

Grounding Techniques for Energy Balance

Grounding practices involve connecting with the Earth's energy to restore balance. Techniques such as walking barefoot on natural surfaces, spending time outdoors, or visualizing roots anchoring into the ground promote a sense of grounding. This holistic approach contributes to emotional stability and overall well-being.

Conclusion

Holistic approaches to well-being encompass a tapestry of practices that harmonize the mind, body, and soul. From mindful movement and meditative practices to energy healing modalities, nutritional considerations, and nature connection, individuals can cultivate a holistic lifestyle that nurtures every facet of their existence. This chapter invites readers to explore the rich landscape of holistic well-being, empowering them to embrace practices that resonate with their unique journey toward a balanced and flourishing life.

Incorporating Practices like Yoga and Meditation

Yoga

In the pursuit of holistic well-being, the incorporation of practices like yoga stands as a transformative journey for the mind, body, and soul. This section explores the multifaceted benefits of yoga, delving into its physical postures, breathwork, and meditative aspects, guiding individuals on a holistic path to wellness.

1. Physical Aspects of Yoga

Asanas for Strength and Flexibility

Yoga asanas, or postures, form the physical foundation of practice. From downward dog to warrior poses, these postures enhance strength, flexibility, and balance. Engaging in a regular yoga routine contributes to improved physical health, supporting joint mobility and muscle tone.

Flowing Movements in Vinyasa Yoga

Vinyasa yoga emphasizes the fluid transition between poses, creating a dynamic and rhythmic flow. The continuous movement synchronizes breath with motion, promoting cardiovascular health, enhancing circulation, and fostering a sense of vitality.

2. Breathwork and Pranayama

Conscious Breath Awareness

Central to yoga is pranayama, or breath control. Practices such as diaphragmatic breathing and ujjayi breathing cultivate conscious breath awareness. This mindful approach to breathing supports relaxation, reduces stress, and anchors the mind in the present moment.

Nadi Shodhana for Balancing Energy Channels

Nadi Shodhana, or alternate nostril breathing, is a pranayama technique that balances the flow of energy in the body. By alternating breath between nostrils, individuals harmonize the left and right sides of the brain, promoting mental clarity and emotional equilibrium.

3. Meditation and Mindfulness

Mindful Meditation Practices

Yoga extends beyond physical postures to embrace meditation. Mindful meditation involves cultivating focused attention on breath, sensations, or a chosen point of focus. Regular meditation sessions contribute to stress reduction, improved concentration, and a heightened sense of inner calm.

Loving-Kindness Meditation (Metta)

Loving-kindness meditation, or Metta, emphasizes cultivating compassion and goodwill toward oneself and others. This practice fosters a positive and open-hearted mindset, promoting emotional resilience and enhancing interpersonal relationships.

4. Yoga Philosophy and Lifestyle Integration

Yamas and Niyamas as Ethical Guidelines

Yoga philosophy encompasses ethical guidelines known as yamas and niyamas. The yamas, including principles like non-violence and truthfulness, offer a moral code for interacting with the external world. The niyamas, such as self-discipline and contentment, provide internal guidelines for personal growth and well-being.

Ahimsa and Compassion in Action

Ahimsa, the principle of non-violence, extends beyond physical harm to include compassion in actions and thoughts. Incorporating ahimsa into daily life fosters a sense of kindness, both towards oneself and others, creating a foundation for holistic well-being.

5. Yoga for Stress Reduction

<u>Restorative Yoga Practices</u>

Restorative yoga focuses on relaxation and rejuvenation. Incorporating supported poses and gentle stretches, restorative yoga activates the parasympathetic nervous system, promoting deep relaxation and stress reduction.

<u>Yoga Nidra for Deep Relaxation</u>

Yoga Nidra, or yogic sleep, is a guided meditation practice that induces a state of deep relaxation. This form of conscious relaxation reduces stress, anxiety, and insomnia, fostering mental and emotional well-being.

6. Personalizing the Yoga Journey

Adapting Yoga to Individual Needs

Holistic well-being through yoga involves personalization. Adapting the practice to individual needs, physical conditions, and preferences ensures a sustainable and enjoyable journey. Whether through gentle yoga, power yoga, or specialized styles, customization enhances the resonance of the practice.

Yoga for Life Transitions

Yoga serves as a supportive tool during life transitions. Whether navigating challenges, transitions, or seeking self-discovery, the holistic nature of yoga offers a space for introspection, resilience-building, and a renewed sense of purpose.

Conclusion

Incorporating practices like yoga unveils a holistic path to well-being, encompassing physical vitality, mental clarity, and emotional balance. The integration of physical postures, breathwork, meditation, and yoga philosophy creates a tapestry of practices that nurture the mind, body, and soul. This chapter invites individuals to embark on a transformative journey, embracing the rich tradition of yoga as a holistic approach to wellness.

Meditation

Meditation, a profound practice with roots in ancient traditions, serves as a transformative journey toward inner harmony and holistic well-being. This section explores the multifaceted benefits of meditation, guiding individuals on the path to cultivating a calm mind, reducing stress, and fostering a deep sense of inner peace.

1. Mindful Meditation Practices

<u>Breath Awareness Meditation</u>

Mindful meditation often begins with breath awareness. By directing attention to the natural rhythm of the breath, individuals cultivate present-moment awareness. This practice promotes relaxation, centers the mind, and serves as a foundational technique for various meditation styles.

<u>Body Scan Meditation</u>

Body scan meditation involves systematically directing attention to different parts of the body, cultivating awareness of sensations. This practice promotes relaxation, releases tension, and enhances the mind-body connection. It is particularly effective for stress reduction and promoting a sense of groundedness.

2. Loving-Kindness Meditation (Metta)

Cultivating Compassion and Goodwill

Loving-kindness meditation, or Metta, focuses on cultivating compassion and goodwill toward oneself and others. Practitioners generate feelings of love, kindness, and compassion, extending these positive intentions to oneself, loved ones, acquaintances, and even those with whom they may have conflicts. Metta meditation enhances emotional well-being and nurtures a compassionate mindset.

Mantra Meditation for Focus

Mantra meditation involves repeating a word, phrase, or sound (mantra) to focus the mind. The rhythmic repetition creates a meditative state, calming the mind and promoting a sense of inner peace. Mantras can be chosen based on personal resonance or spiritual significance.

3. Transcendental Meditation (TM)

Effortless Transcendence

Transcendental Meditation, founded by Maharishi Mahesh Yogi, involves the silent repetition of a specific mantra. TM is characterized by its simplicity and effortlessness, allowing the mind to transcend ordinary thought and experience a state of deep restful awareness. This practice is associated with reduced stress and increased clarity of thought.

Mindfulness-Based Stress Reduction (MBSR)

Mindfulness-Based Stress Reduction (MBSR) is a structured program that incorporates mindfulness meditation to reduce stress and enhance well-being. Developed by Dr. Jon Kabat-Zinn, MBSR combines mindfulness meditation, yoga, and awareness practices to promote stress resilience and improve mental health.

4. Zen Meditation (Zazen)

<u>Silent Sitting Meditation</u>

Zen meditation, or Zazen, is a form of seated meditation rooted in Zen Buddhism. Practitioners sit in a specific posture, focusing on the breath and observing thoughts without attachment. Zazen aims to cultivate a deep awareness of the present moment, fostering inner stillness and insight.

Walking Meditation for Movement

Walking meditation combines mindfulness with the act of walking. Practitioners focus on the sensations of walking, the movement of the body, and the surrounding environment. This dynamic meditation allows individuals to cultivate mindfulness while engaging in a rhythmic and purposeful activity.

5. Guided Imagery and Visualization

Creative Visualization

Guided imagery and visualization involve creating mental images or scenarios to evoke positive sensations and emotions. Guided by a teacher or through recorded sessions, individuals engage their imagination to promote relaxation, reduce stress, and enhance overall well-being.

Journeying Through Mental Landscapes

Guided meditation journeys invite individuals to mentally explore specific landscapes or scenarios. Whether a peaceful beach, a forest, or an imaginary world, these journeys promote relaxation, creativity, and a sense of inner exploration.

6. Mindfulness in Daily Activities

Mindful Eating

Mindful eating involves bringing full attention to the experience of eating. By savoring flavors, textures, and aromas, individuals cultivate a deep appreciation for nourishment, reduce overeating, and foster a healthier relationship with food.

Mindful Walking and Movement

Mindfulness extends to daily activities, including walking and movement. By bringing awareness to each step, the rhythm of movement, and the sensations in the body, individuals integrate mindfulness into their daily routines, promoting a sense of presence and calm.

Conclusion

Incorporating practices like meditation offers a gateway to inner harmony and holistic well-being. Whether through mindful meditation, loving-kindness practices, or visualization, individuals can choose methods that resonate with their preferences and goals. This chapter invites you to embark on a journey of self-discovery, exploring the transformative power of meditation in cultivating a calm and centered mind.

Chapter 10

Beyond Recovery

Chapter 10 marks the transition from recovery to a renewed chapter of life—one that extends beyond the challenges of binge eating. As we delve into "Beyond Recovery," this section illuminates the path forward, addressing the nuances of navigating relapses and setbacks with resilience. Emphasis is placed on cultivating a positive relationship with food, inviting readers to embrace a future where well-being and a harmonious connection with nourishment become the cornerstones of a fulfilling life.

This chapter dives into:

1. Life After Binge Eating

★ Navigating Relapses and Setbacks

★ Cultivating a Positive Relationship with Food

Life After Binge Eating

In the aftermath of the intense journey through recovery, Chapter 10 ushers in a new phase—"Life After Binge Eating." Here, the narrative transcends the confines of disorder, offering a glimpse into a liberated existence where individuals rediscover joy, embrace newfound freedom, and navigate the uncharted terrain of post-recovery with resilience and optimism. As we embark on this chapter, the focus shifts from overcoming challenges to savoring the possibilities that await on the path to a fulfilling and nourished life.

Navigating Relapses and Setbacks

The journey toward recovery from binge eating is a path marked by progress, self-discovery, and, inevitably, moments of challenge. In Chapter 10, "Navigating Relapses and Setbacks," we delve into the nuanced terrain of setbacks, offering insights, strategies, and a compassionate perspective to guide individuals through moments that may test their resolve on the road to healing.

1. Understanding the Nature of Setbacks

Normalizing the Ebb and Flow

Setbacks are a natural part of the recovery journey. It's crucial to understand that occasional relapses or setbacks do not diminish the progress made. The journey to overcome binge eating is characterized by peaks and valleys, and setbacks provide valuable opportunities for learning and growth.

Identifying Triggers and Patterns

Examining the circumstances surrounding setbacks is essential for understanding triggers and patterns. By identifying specific situations, emotions, or stressors that contribute to setbacks, individuals can develop targeted strategies to address these challenges and enhance their resilience.

2. Building Resilience in the Face of Setbacks

Cultivating Self-Compassion

Self-compassion is a powerful tool during setbacks. Rather than succumbing to self-criticism, individuals can cultivate self-compassion by acknowledging their struggles with kindness and understanding. This mindset shift fosters resilience and a more positive relationship with oneself.

Learning from Setbacks

Setbacks provide valuable insights into areas that may need further attention or support. By approaching setbacks as learning opportunities, individuals can extract valuable information about their triggers, coping mechanisms, and areas for growth, contributing to a more resilient recovery process.

3. Reconnecting with Support Systems

Seeking Professional Guidance

During setbacks, seeking support from mental health professionals can be instrumental. Therapists, counselors, and support groups offer tailored guidance and tools to navigate challenges. Professional support provides a safe space to explore the underlying factors contributing to setbacks and develop effective coping strategies.

Engaging with Peer Support

Peer support plays a vital role in resilience. Connecting with others who have experienced similar challenges fosters a sense of shared understanding and encouragement. Online communities, support groups, or recovery networks provide avenues for individuals to share experiences and receive empathetic support.

4. **Adjusting and Refining Strategies**

Reassessing and Modifying Goals

Setbacks may prompt a reassessment of recovery goals. It's essential to approach this process with flexibility and openness. Modifying goals based on current circumstances, priorities, and insights gained from setbacks ensures that the recovery journey remains realistic and sustainable.

Refining Coping Mechanisms

Exploring and refining coping mechanisms is an ongoing process. Setbacks offer an opportunity to evaluate the effectiveness of existing strategies and explore additional tools for managing stress, emotions, and triggers. This adaptive approach contributes to enhanced resilience.

5. Mindful Reflection and Planning Ahead

Reflecting on Progress

Taking time for mindful reflection on overall progress is crucial. Recognizing the achievements and positive changes made during the recovery journey reinforces resilience. Acknowledging personal growth provides motivation and a sense of accomplishment.

Developing a Relapse Prevention Plan

A relapse prevention plan is a proactive tool for navigating potential setbacks. By collaboratively developing strategies with mental health professionals, individuals can outline specific steps to take when faced with triggers or challenging situations. This personalized plan empowers individuals to respond effectively and maintain progress.

Conclusion

In the realm of recovery, setbacks are not roadblocks but rather stepping stones to resilience and continued growth. Chapter 10, "Navigating Relapses and Setbacks," encourages individuals to approach challenges with self-compassion, seek support, and view setbacks as opportunities for learning and refinement. By incorporating these insights and strategies, individuals can navigate the complexities of recovery with resilience, fostering a sense of empowerment on their path to healing.

Cultivating a Positive Relationship with Food

In the final stretch of the recovery journey, Chapter 10 invites individuals to explore the transformative practice of cultivating a positive relationship with food. This section emphasizes the importance of fostering a healthy and mindful connection with nourishment, moving beyond the shadows of binge eating towards a balanced, joyful, and sustainable approach to eating.

1. Understanding the Foundations of Positive Eating

<u>Mindful Eating Principles</u>

Mindful eating serves as the cornerstone of a positive relationship with food. This practice involves being fully present during meals, savoring flavors, and paying attention to hunger and fullness cues. By approaching eating with intention and awareness, individuals can develop a more gratifying and mindful connection with their meals.

<u>Honoring Hunger and Fullness</u>

Listening to the body's signals of hunger and fullness is fundamental. Cultivating an awareness of physical cues helps individuals reconnect with their internal regulatory mechanisms, promoting a balanced and intuitive approach to eating.

2. Challenging Food Myths and Dichotomies

Breaking Free from Good vs. Bad Mentality

Cultivating a positive relationship with food requires challenging ingrained beliefs about "good" and "bad" foods. Instead of adopting restrictive or dichotomous thinking, individuals can embrace a more inclusive and flexible mindset that allows for a diverse and satisfying range of foods.

Addressing Food Guilt and Shame

Guilt and shame surrounding food choices can hinder progress. This section encourages individuals to address and reframe negative emotions associated with eating. Developing self-compassion and understanding that food is not a moral compass but a source of nourishment fosters a positive mindset.

3. Exploring Pleasure and Satisfaction in Eating

Savoring Food Experiences

Cultivating a positive relationship with food involves savoring the sensory aspects of eating. Whether it's appreciating the aroma, texture, or taste of a meal, focusing on the pleasure of eating enhances the overall dining experience and contributes to a positive association with food.

Balancing Nutritional Needs and Enjoyment

Balancing nutritional needs with the enjoyment of food is a key principle. This involves incorporating a variety of nutrient-dense foods while also allowing space for foods that bring joy and satisfaction. The integration of both aspects contributes to a sustainable and positive eating pattern.

4. Building Skills for Intuitive Eating

Developing Intuitive Eating Practices

Intuitive eating involves attuning to the body's natural hunger and fullness cues. By developing this skill, individuals can move away from external rules or diets, fostering a more intuitive and harmonious relationship with food based on internal cues.

Practicing Mindful Food Choices

Mindful food choices involve considering the nutritional and emotional aspects of food. This practice encourages individuals to make food choices that align with both physical well-being and personal preferences, contributing to a positive and balanced eating experience.

5. Creating a Supportive Food Environment

Surrounding Oneself with Positive Influences

Building a positive food environment involves surrounding oneself with supportive influences. This may include connecting with individuals who share similar positive eating goals, engaging in supportive communities, and seeking encouragement from friends, family, or professionals.

Minimizing Triggering Factors

Identifying and minimizing triggering factors in the food environment is crucial. This may involve creating a home environment that aligns with positive eating goals, reducing exposure to diet culture, and establishing boundaries that support a nurturing relationship with food.

6. Mindful Meal Planning and Preparation

Engaging in Joyful Cooking and Meal Preparation

Transforming meal planning and preparation into joyful activities contributes to a positive relationship with food. By exploring new recipes, experimenting with flavors, and involving oneself in the cooking process, individuals can infuse meals with creativity and enjoyment.

Balancing Structure and Flexibility

Balancing structure and flexibility in meal planning promotes a positive approach. While having a basic structure provides a sense of routine, allowing flexibility accommodates changing preferences and spontaneous enjoyment, creating a sustainable and positive eating rhythm.

Conclusion

Cultivating a positive relationship with food is a transformative journey that extends beyond recovery. Chapter 10 encourages individuals to embrace mindful and intuitive eating, challenge restrictive thinking, and foster a balanced, joy-filled approach to nourishment. By incorporating these principles, individuals can embark on a path where food becomes a source of nourishment, pleasure, and empowerment, contributing to a sustained and positive well-being.

Conclusion

As we bid farewell to the pages that unfolded the tapestry of your journey within **"Transform Beyond the Buffet: Unraveling the Complexities of Binge Eating,"** let this conclusion be a rallying cry, an anthem that echoes in the corridors of your newfound empowerment. The journey is far from over; it's a living, breathing practice that awaits your daily embrace.

It's about embracing the insights, strategies, and wisdom woven into the fabric of these book. Your practice is the crucible where transformation occurs, where knowledge turns into wisdom, and where each intentional step becomes a stride toward a life free from the shadows of binge eating.

In the hustle and bustle of life, it's easy to lose sight of the why that ignited this journey. As you navigate the intricacies of your practice, take a moment to honor the reason you embarked on this path. Your why is the compass that guides you through challenges, a North Star reminding you of the profound transformation you seek. In the daily grind, let your why be the unwavering heartbeat that propels you forward.

Your journey is not yours alone; it's a torch that can illuminate the paths of others. As you practice and witness the blossoming of your own resilience, consider sharing your light. Extend a helping hand, lend a compassionate ear, or simply be a beacon of hope for someone navigating the labyrinth of binge eating. Your story is a powerful instrument of inspiration, a testament that recovery is possible, and a beacon that can guide others out of the darkness.

Your words have power—they can spark motivation, instill hope, and guide fellow travelers on their journeys. If this book has resonated with you, consider dropping a review. Share your thoughts, your insights, and the transformations you've experienced. Your review is not just feedback; it's a ripple that can create waves of change, reaching those who may need it the most.

As you step away from these pages, remember that your journey is ongoing. Every practice session, every reflection, and every choice you make is a brushstroke on the canvas of your vibrant life. Keep practicing, honor your why, share your light, and let the echoes of your transformation resound in the tapestry of your future.

May your days be filled with the strength of practice, the clarity of purpose, and the radiant glow of a life unfettered by binge eating. Your journey is an inspiration, and your story is a beacon—may it shine brightly for you and for others.

With gratitude and the anticipation of your continued success,

[Unique Kade]

www.ingramcontent.com/pod-product-compliance
Lightning Source LLC
Chambersburg PA
CBHW070920260726
48661CB00003B/768